Intermittent Fasting for Women over 50

A Comprehensive Guide to Lose Weight, Challenge Aging, Revitalize Energy and Achieve Hormonal Balance for Lifelong Health and Confidence

CARMEN THIES

DEDICATION

I would like to dedicate this book to all women who have struggled at some point in their lives with feeling young, vital, and healthy. To those who see the need and strive for change for the better, and to those who are ready to claim power over their health, bodies, and lives.

You are never alone and never will be

CONTENTS

PREFACE

Greetings from a life-changing adventure that reinterprets what health, age, and vitality really mean. As a nutritionist, nurse, and midwife, my commitment to women's health has motivated me to investigate the many advantages of intermittent fasting, an age-old but surprisingly cutting-edge scientific practice. My own and my work experiences with this amazing approach are the basis for this book. I found in intermittent fasting not just a diet but a dramatic lifestyle transformation, having personally battled with binge-eating and the difficulties of maintaining optimal health in a hectic medical career. It has transformed my attitude on food, restored my energy, and brought me my health back.

This isn't just another guide; it's a testament to the transformative power of intermittent fasting, particularly for women over 50 who are navigating the complex changes of menopause. From hormonal shifts to metabolism adjustments, intermittent fasting offers a tailored solution that promotes rejuvenation at a cellular level. This book is crafted with both passion and knowledge, aiming to empower you to reclaim control over your health and vitality.

Welcome to your new beginning!

ACKNOWLEDGMENTS

I want to express my deepest gratitude to all the women who shared their personal stories and inspired this book—thank you for your courage, honesty, and wisdom. This book would not have been possible without your contributions

INTRODUCTION

This book offers comprehensive guidance created especially for women over 50, aimed at maximizing the benefits of intermittent fasting to address specific health requirements and revitalize the body and mind. It clarifies intermittent fasting with a focus on how it can be modified to promote hormone balance, energy restoration, and general health renewal in addition to weight loss.

The scientific foundations of intermittent fasting, including its effects on hormones and metabolism, will be covered. From getting started on your intermittent fasting adventure to smoothly incorporating it into your daily routine, each chapter offers helpful guidance. You'll discover in-depth explanations of how intermittent fasting can be your ally against the aging process as well as inspirational insights to keep you motivated.

As we explore the chapters, you will find specific techniques that take into account your body's requirements, providing a sustainable way of living rather than merely a diet. This book tries to provide you all the tools you need to start along this path that can improve your life, regardless of your level of experience with dietary modifications or your familiarity with fasting, and includes import worksheets that help you along your way.

1 UNDERSTANDING INTERMITTENT FASTING

Definition and Benefits of Intermittent Fasting

A pattern of eating known as intermittent fasting alternates times of eating and fasting. Intermittent fasting focusses on *when* you eat rather than *what* you consume, as do conventional diets. It lays out times when you should eat and fast rather than prescribing certain foods or calorie counts. Eating this way can help you lose weight, have better metabolic health, and even live longer.

Fundamentally, intermittent fasting is a strategy meant to signal the body to release stored energy, which increases metabolic efficiency and energy use. Just as crucial as reducing calories is allowing the body the time it needs to repair, renew, and optimize its internal functions without the ongoing demands of digestion. During this fast, the body can retrain its insulin response, help break down fat stores more effectively for energy, and regulate hormones.

All adults can benefit from intermittent fasting because it is highly adaptable and can be made to fit individual objectives and way of life. The next chapters will discuss several types of intermittent fasting and which ones are ideal for women over 50. Better results will come from the right form of intermittent fasting being chosen by instinct depending on the goal, physical attributes, work/rest balance, and life circumstances. Though it is up to you, I advise you to consult with your healthcare provider if you have any serious medical issues or are unsure about the best kind of intermittent fasting for you.

The Historical Journey and Global Popularity of Intermittent Fasting

Intermittent fasting has always been an element of spiritual rituals, culture, and human evolution. The roots of it are found in prehistoric societies. Fasting used to be usually a decision rather than the outcome of food shortage. Our ancestors developed physiological adaptations to this feast-or-famine mode of life in order to survive during times of food scarcity. This evolutionary characteristic raises the prospect that our natural biological rhythms and periodic fasting are closely related.

Going back beyond its accidental use in prehistoric times, fasting has been actively practiced for physical health, mental clarity, and spiritual cleansing throughout a wide spectrum of cultures and religions. Philosophers of antiquity such as Socrates, Plato, and Hippocrates praised the virtues of fasting and connected it to longer life and better cognitive performance. In the same way, fasting is included into the rituals of all major religions: Christianity, Islam, Judaism, Buddhism, and Hinduism.

The 20th-century scientific literature started to publish the contemporary, health- and wellness-focused version of intermittent fasting. Still, the public and medical community did not pay intermittent fasting much attention until the twenty-first century. This comeback has been credited to new studies showing its possible advantages over and above basic weight loss, such as longer lifespans, better metabolic health, and lower risk factors for a number of chronic illnesses.

In recent years, intermittent fasting has become incredibly popular thanks in large part to social media, celebrity endorsements, and scientific evidence. As digital technology expanded, practitioners have found it simpler to get together globally and promote intermittent fasting as a long-term lifestyle choice as opposed to a temporary diet.

Though intermittent fasting has historical roots, its appeal today is a testament to its flexibility and continuous quest for the best methods for health and wellbeing. Intermittent fasting is an intriguing combination of traditional beliefs and contemporary science that appeals to anyone seeking a comprehensive approach to health in a world that is changing and moving more quickly than ever.

The Science Behind Intermittent Fasting: Autophagy and Its Discovery

Intermittent fasting has drawn a lot of interest because of its metabolic and weight-loss benefits as well as its deeper biological impacts, particularly in terms of boosting autophagy. The Greek terms for "self" (auto) and "eating" (phagy) are where the phrase "self-eating," or autophagy, originates. A key process in preserving cellular health and function, this cellular mechanism involves th body's systematic degradation and recycling of cellular components.

When researching insulin in the 1960s, Belgian biochemist Christian de Duve is credited with developing autophagy and its mechanics. De Duve's groundbreaking study won him the 1974 Nobel Prize in Physiology or Medicine. The 2016 Nobel Prize in Physiology or Medicine was to Yoshinori Ohsumi for his further 1990s study that clarified the genes required for autophagy. The basic ideas of autophagy were explained and its importance for many physiological processes, including starvation and infection response, was demonstrated by Ohsumi's study on yeast cells.

Because the body needs more energy during fasting periods than it can obtain from food, it shifts its energy metabolism from glucose to ketosis and activates autophagic pathways. It takes this process to maintain cellular renewal, fight cellular stress, and remove damaged cellular components. By doing this, autophagy makes it possible to avoid diseases caused by aging and cellular breakdown, such as infections, cancer, and neurological disorders.

Nowadays, new insights on human health and disease are emerging as research on autophagy and intermittent fasting progress, showing the important impact of dietary habits on the fundamental biological functions of our bodies.

Important Process of Mitophagy

Mitophagy is a specific type of autophagy, which is an essential cellular mechanism that involves the degradation and recycling of cellular constituents. More specifically, mitochondria are degraded selectively via mitophagy. It's common to refer to mitochondria as the cell's power plants. These are specialized organelles that are present in the majority of eukaryotic organisms' cells. They are in charge of cellular respiration, the mechanism by which ATP (adenosine triphosphate) is produced. Apart from generating energy, mitochondria are engaged in various other functions such as signaling, cellular differentiation, cell death, regulation of the cell cycle, and cell growth.

Particularly important is the process of mitophagy in tissues with high energy requirements, such as the brain and heart. Diseases such as metabolic disorders, cardiovascular diseases, general tissue aging, and neurodegenerative diseases like Parkinson's and Alzheimer's have all been related to impairments in mitophagy.

The DNA contained in mitochondria is different from that found in the cell nucleus, making mitochondria unique. This mitochondrial DNA is passed on from mothers to their offspring and permits the production of certain proteins required for the mitochondria's proper operation. Healthy mitochondria are essential for preserving overall cellular and body health because of their crucial role in producing energy and controlling cellular metabolism.

The Role of Mitophagy

ing defective or damaged mitochondria, mitophagy helps o cellular health by reducing the production of excess reactive es (ROS), which may otherwise result in oxidative stress and ige. Mitophagy plays an important part in maintaining cellular energy production, which is vital to the health and longevity of cells, by controlling the quantity and quality of mitochondria. Increased oxidative stress, which accelerates cellular aging and is linked to chronic diseases like diabetes and cardiovascular disease—diseases that are more common in postmenopausal women—is caused by aged and inefficient mitochondria.

In order to sustain mitochondrial synthesis and provide protection against oxidative stress, estrogen plays a part in influencing mitochondrial activity. Menopause-related decrease in estrogen may reduce mitochondrial activity, which causes energy depletion and increases sensitivity to oxidative damage.

Mitophagy and Intermittent Fasting

According to recent studies, intermittent fasting may improve mitophagy, which in turn may aid in cellular renewal and repair. Mitophagy is triggered by a variety of metabolic processes and stress responses that are brought on by fasting. This enhances mitochondrial function and aids in the detoxification of cells from damaged mitochondria, which may increase longevity and energy efficiency.

Key Mechanism of Intermittent Fasting: Synchronizing Biological Rhythms

Intermittent fasting is primarily driven by the biological cycles of the body that control eating and fasting cycles. It takes this synchronization to increase metabolic functions, raise health results, and possibly prolong life.

These are the main intermittent fasting mechanisms:

Activation of Metabolic Switches

Intermittent fasting causes the body to switch metabolically from creating energy from glucose to ketone bodies. The body enters ketosis, or this shift, when it runs out of glycogen and starts using fat for energy. Along with being essential for weight loss, this metabolic change also significantly contributes to reduced inflammation, improved memory, and longer life.

Enhancement of Autophagy

Mostly because it initiates autophagy, the body's cellular cleansing mechanism, intermittent fasting is good for health. As was already indicated, maintaining cellular function, helping with cellular repair, and removing damaged proteins and cells depend on autophagy. It is essential to postpone aging and has been linked to a reduced risk of certain chronic diseases.

Improvement in Hormonal Balance

The regulation of hormones is greatly affected by intermittent fasting. Improving insulin sensitivity assures that cells respond to insulin more effectively, which helps to regulate glucose and reduces the chance of type 2 diabetes. Moreover, fasting affects leptin and ghrelin, two other hormones associated with hunger and satiety, which helps regulate appetite and prevent overeating.

Strengthening of Circadian Rhythms

The body's circadian rhythms—natural, internal processes that control the sleep-wake cycle and recur about every 24 hours—are strengthened by intermittent fasts. By following these rhythms—eating during the day and fasting at night—one can improve metabolic health, sleep quality, and daily alertness. Supporting the body's natural processes, this synchronization enhances general health.

Reduction of Inflammation and Oxidative Stress

Intermittent fasting lowers inflammation and oxidative stress in the body by prolonging fasting times and reducing meal frequency. These advantages are vital for shielding against chronic illnesses including heart disease, cancer, and neurological diseases as well as age-related deterioration.

Enhancement of Brain Health

Intermittent fasting has advantages for the brain, including neurogenesis—the growth of new neurons—and enhanced resistance to stress and injury. One way these effects are mediated is by increased synthesis of the protein brain-derived neurotrophic factor (BDNF), which enhances brain plasticity and cognitive performance.

Effects on Levels of HGH, or Human Growth Hormone

A key hormone released by the pituitary gland, HGH has a major effect on growth, body composition, cell repair, and metabolism. Studies show that fasting increases HGH, which helps grow muscle, reduce fat, and heal from injuries. This rise in HGH throughout fasting periods supports the body's ability to preserve lean muscle mass and also encourages the burning of fat for energy, therefore enhancing metabolic health and body composition.

Gene Expression

Intermittent fasting affects gene expression and opens up pathways that extend life and protect against illness. Intermittent fasting can start cellular processes that improve stress resilience, slow down aging, and lower the risk of chronic diseases by influencing the expression of genes associated to metabolism, stress resistance, and repair mechanisms. These genetic alterations demonstrate the significant effects of fasting on cellular function and general health and the possibility of dietary treatments to regulate gene expression for better health results.

Exploring the Types of Intermittent Fasting

Intermittent fasting offers a versatile approach to eating that can be adapted to fit various lifestyles, preferences, and health goals. Here, we explore eight popular types of intermittent fasting, each with its unique structure and potential benefits.

The 16/8 Method

By this approach, one fasts for sixteen hours a day and eats inside an eight-hour window. Those who are new to intermittent fasting will find it to be one of the more popular and doable types. This approach is easier as it looks because night sleep covers over half of those 16 hours.

The 5:2 Diet

Those that follow this kind of intermittent fasting eat normally five days a week and drastically cut back on calories on two non-consecutive days, usually to 500–600. Rather than requiring total fasting, this method concentrates on calorie reduction.

Eat-Stop-Eat

This is a whole 24-hour fast, either once or twice a week. It's a more difficult schedule that calls for fasting from dinner one day to dinner the following.

Alternative-Day Fasting (ADF)

Days when you either fast entirely or consume a very low-calorie intake (approximately 500 calories) alternate with days when you eat normally. Beginners might not be appropriate for this more demanding method.

The Warrior Diet

With the Warrior Diet, one eats a big dinner at night within a 4-hour eating window and little amounts of raw fruits and vegetables during the day, therefore fasting for 20 hours every day.

The 12/12 Method

This approach divides the day into equal 12-hour eating and fasting intervals, making intermittent a milder start. Those who wish to experiment with intermittent fasting without making major lifestyle adjustments will find it especially helpful. If you would want to implement the 16/8 Method, you can start with this and gradually increase the fasting hours from 12 to 14 and 16.

The OMAD Diet (One Meal a Day)

One extreme type of fasting called OMAD involves eating all of your daily calories in one meal and then fasting the remainder of the day. Meeting your nutritional demands all at once is important for a well-planned lunch.

Spontaneous Meal Skipping

Rather than stetting a fasting schedule, this method entails skipping meals when it's practical. This adaptable approach supports intuitive eating and stresses eating only when really hungry, but keeping the food amounts healthy.

Which Types Work Best for Women Over 50?

The best intermittent fasting methods for women over 50 are those that help to maintain hormonal balance, efficiently control weight, and do not excessively stress the body. Excellent starting points, the 16/8 and 12/12 methods provide a reasonable fasting period that fits with regular daily rhythms. These techniques are easily modified to suit into an active, healthy lifestyle and are less prone to upset hormone balance.

Additionally appropriate is the 5:2 Diet, which provides the advantages of calorie restriction while allowing for regular eating most days of the week. Without the everyday dedication to a strict fasting window, this approach can help control weight and enhance metabolic health.

You will find that the best approach depends in the long run on your particular lifestyle, health goals, and body's response to fasting. If you can't decide which method is best for you, start with the 16/8 Method or work your way up from the 12/12 Method. Results will ultimately show up, even though they might not do so immediately.

2 STARTING YOUR INTERMITTENT FASTING JOURNEY

Welcome to the most exciting chapter! Starting an intermittent fasting is the first step on a transformative journey toward better health, more energy, and a greater awareness of your body's demands. It's so important to set reasonable goals, monitor your progress, choose a fasting regimen that fits your lifestyle, and both mentally and physically prepare for a successful and long-lasting practice. You will receive guidance through fundamental steps in this chapter, giving you the knowledge and resources, you need to confidently start your process.

Preparing Mentally and Physically for Your Intermittent Fasting Journey

Mental Preparation

To be at the point where you are now, reading this book – shows that you are mentally ready to accept the benefits of intermittent fasting. Probably you are also ready to step in. Maybe even some of the steps for mental preparation already lie behind and you are curious and impatient to start. Still, I encourage you to read through these simple bits of advice.

Educate Yourself

Begin by deepening your understanding of intermittent fasting. Research its mechanisms, benefits, and potential challenges. Knowledge is empowering and can help dispel any apprehensions or misconceptions you might have. One way to educate yourself is to speak with people who tried or integrated intermittent fasting into their lives, so you can learn from their experience.

Set Your Intentions

Reflect on why you're starting intermittent fasting. Is it for weight loss, improved mental clarity, or longevity? Understanding your motivation provides a clear direction and keeps you focused during tough times. There is a famous saying, stating that a child learns from example, and the adult learns from self-reflection. Many, if not all, of physical problems are related to our emotions and mental condition. And by reflecting on them we come to a point of clarity, which can be beneficial in making the issues disappear or become less disturbing.

Cultivate a Positive Mindset

Adopt a positive and flexible mindset! View intermittent fasting as a journey of self-discovery and health improvement. Recognize that there will be challenges and learning curves, but with resilience and adaptability, you can overcome them. Trust yourself and don't blame yourself if there will be no fast results or days when something goes unplanned.

Be open about your journey

Inform your friends or family, who are close to you and may influence your diet and food intake and preparation. In my case it was the most difficult thing to do: to tell my colleagues at work, why I didn't have breakfast. There were mixed opinions on the matter, some of them were judgmental, but others supported and started to share their stories about intermittent fasting. Our community can be ruthless sometimes, but it also can be extremely supportive when we need it.

Manage Stress

High stress can sabotage your intermittent fasting efforts, affecting your ability to stick to fasting periods and make healthy food choices. Find stress-reduction techniques that work for you, such as meditation, yoga, or deep-breathing exercises. It can be easier said than done, but consider this advice as the most important life skill. Stress is closely connected to our nutritional habits – some people skip food or eat unhealthily; some consume too much to soothe their emotions and stress. I remember my worst evenings, as I was coming back from my shift in the hospital, opening the fridge and eating everything I could find there. I ate with two awful feelings inside me: the ache in my stomach and the self-blame in my soul. Fortunately, intermittent fasting, combined with stress management, helped me to cure this condition totally.

Physical Preparation

Health Check-Up

Before starting intermittent fasting, it's advisable to consult with a healthcare provider, especially if you have underlying health conditions. This step ensures that intermittent fasting is safe and suitable for you. Especially ask about which type is more considerable for you. In case the healthcare provider lets this choice on you, I recommend aiming for the 16/8 Method.

Nutritional Adjustment

Aim to incorporate full, nutrient-dense foods into your diet gradually so that it will sustain your body during periods of fasting. Cut back on processed meals, sweets, and too much caffeine as they might aggravate hunger and energy swings.. The best thing to do is to declutter your kitchen and review your fridge: that way you will not be disturbed in your journey. With time your cravings for sweets and unhealthy food will reduce and you will be able to look at them with neutral feelings.

Hydration

Proper hydration is crucial, especially during fasting periods. Water, herbal teas, and electrolyte-rich beverages can help maintain hydration levels without breaking your fast. Further, we will discuss the importance of hydration in Chapter 3.

Sleep Quality

Ensure you are getting enough restful sleep. Poor sleep can affect your hunger hormones, making fasting more challenging and potentially leading to unhealthy eating patterns during your eating windows. As you already can imagine, sleep quality increases as you practice intermittent fasting – and it has a positive effect on stress relief and feeling vital and full of power. My acupuncture practitioner told me every time I was having a session, that from the perspective of Traditional Chinese Medicine sleep is the remedy number one. No healing and no changes for the better can happen, if there is no healthy, sufficient sleep. But the best thing about intermittent fasting is, that it helps to regulate the sleeping pattern which results in better night rest.

Gentle Transition

If you're new to intermittent fasting, consider starting with less restrictive fasting methods, such as the 12/12 Method, and gradually increase your fasting window. This approach allows your body and mind to adjust without overwhelming stress.

Physical Activity and Exercise

Incorporate regular physical activity into your routine, tailored to your fitness level. Exercise can enhance the effects of intermittent fasting, improving body composition and metabolic health. However, listen to your body and adjust the intensity and timing of workouts to complement your fasting and feeding cycles. Physical activity is every activity that could boost your metabolism, may it be walking, house cleaning, or dancing. In Chapter 6 we will discuss the importance of physical activity more closely.

You may create a strong foundation for your journey into intermittent fasting by emotionally and physically preparing yourself sufficiently. This optimizes the advantages of this successful lifestyle approach and facilitates the transition to intermittent fasting. It's important to remember that developing healthy habits over time will affect your relationship with food and increase your awareness of your body's needs. You can make it!

Choosing the Right Method

Which intermittent fasting strategy you choose to use can make a major difference in how successful and enjoyable your fasting experience is. With so many options, it's important to comprehend how the small variations in tactics relate to your individual lifestyle, health objectives, and dietary requirements. This section provides recommendations to assist you in selecting the most appropriate intermittent fasting method. At the end of the book, you will find a worksheet for helping you to make your choice.

Consider Your Lifestyle

The first step in choosing the right intermittent fasting method involves a careful assessment of your daily routine, work demands, social commitments, and personal preferences.

Work and Sleep Patterns

Consider your work hours and sleep schedule. If you have a traditional 9-5 job, a fasting method like the 16/8 Method, where you skip breakfast but eat lunch and dinner, might fit very well into your day. Alternatively, if you work night shifts, you may need to adapt your fasting window to align with your unconventional schedule. As a medical worker in the hospital, I chose this method and it was a perfect fit for my always changing work schedule. In fact, I was able to regulate the eating times during night shifts and it played a big role in weight loss and eliminating the stress dependent binge-eating.

Social and Family Commitments

Think about your social life and family meals. If dinner is an important family gathering you don't want to miss, ensure your eating window accommodates this. The flexibility of the fasting schedule can be crucial for long-term commitment.

Align with Your Health Goals

Your health and fitness objectives play a crucial role in determining the most suitable method. Let as explore the most popular goals for intermittent fasting and what impact it has on body.

Weight Loss

If your primary goal is weight loss, longer fasting periods, such as the 20/4 Warrior Diet or OMAD, may offer faster results. These methods significantly restrict your eating window, potentially reducing your overall calorie intake. However, the jo-jo effect may be more possible by practicing those methods and they are not suitable for people with severe health conditions, as well as for those taking medications. In my opinion, the best weight loss is a slow, but steady process that can be easy to keep up. In this case, the desired weight is also kept better without much effort and weight fluctuations.

Metabolic Health

For improving metabolic health, such as better blood sugar control or increased insulin sensitivity, methods like the 16/8 or the 5:2 diet can be effective without being overly restrictive. If you have problems with blood sugar levels, please consult with a healthcare provider before starting with intermittent fasting. In some cases, the longest fasting break is allowed to be around 12 hours, but eventually, the breaks can grow longer when blood sugar levels become more stable.

Lifestyle Diseases

Many health conditions play a role in choosing the right method for intermittent fasting. Some of them are hypertension, thyroid issues, increased stomach acidity, and, for example, postoperative period of restoration. In this case, the approach should be delicate and individual, because those methods are not "one size fits all". Generally, intermittent fasting has no side effects, if done correctly according to your body's needs. On the other side, individually, some side effects may arise. This can happen due to several reasons: pushing the body too hard; not being prepared mentally and physically; choosing the wrong method; and not considering health conditions and diagnosis.

If you start with intermittent fasting, your goal will always be having a positive outcome: that's why it is crucial to adjust your method according to your health issues, to avoid more severe damage and deepening of those damages.

Assess Your Dietary Needs

Understanding your nutritional requirements and eating habits is essential when choosing an intermittent fasting method.

Nutrient Intake

Ensure that the intermittent fasting method you choose allows adequate intake of essential nutrients. Further we will discuss special nutrient needs in Chapter 3.

Eating Preferences

If you prefer larger, less frequent meals, a method with a shorter eating window (like OMAD) might suit you. If you enjoy smaller, more frequent meals, a longer eating window (such as the 16/8 Method) may be more sustainable.

Experiment and Adapt

Finding the right intermittent fasting method may require experimentation. Start with a method that seems most compatible with your lifestyle and goals, and be prepared to adjust based on your experiences. Maybe after some time, you will come to a point when you can combine different methods and feel amazing about finding YOUR method.

Trial Period

Give yourself a trial period with a chosen method to monitor how your body and mind respond. Some adaptation challenges are normal, but persistent issues may indicate a need for adjustment. You will find worksheets for self-reflection at the end of this book. Alternatively, you can use the diary to write down some of the changes and body/mind experiences that will help you to adapt even better with time.

Listen to Your Body

Pay attention to your body's signals. If you feel excessively tired, or hungry, or if your performance at work or in workouts declines, consider modifying your fasting method or consulting a healthcare professional. In some cases, the period to start intermittent fasting is not suitable for the body and/or life conditions: for example, after surgery or trauma, or in times of grief.

In conclusion, choosing the right intermittent fasting method is a highly personal decision that should consider your lifestyle, health goals, and dietary needs. There is no "one size fits all" approach, and what works for one person may not work for another. By carefully considering these factors and being open to adjusting your approach, you can find an intermittent fasting method that not only fits your life but enhances your health and wellbeing.

Setting Realistic Goals and Expectations

How to set goals

It is very important to note that not every goal is achievable. In many cases, it is a fact: and not because of a lack of motivation, dedication, discipline, etc.

Very often is the goal just far from realistic and achievable. For example, if your weight loss goal is 25 pounds a month, it could be very difficult to achieve and possibly the whole process will be damaging to your physical and mental health. If you need some advice on how to set realistic goals, try the SMART Method.

The SMART method is a widely used framework for setting clear and achievable goals. Each letter in "SMART" stands for a specific criterion that helps ensure goals are well-defined and reachable:

Specific: Goals should be clear and specific, so you know exactly what you're aiming to achieve (For example, I want to lose 10 pounds and improve my blood sugar levels by practicing the 16/8 intermittent fasting method).

Measurable: Goals should have criteria that allow you to track your progress and measure success (For example, I will track weight loss through regular weigh-ins and monitor blood sugar levels through medical tests).

Achievable: Goals should be realistic and attainable to be successful (Losing 10 pounds and improving blood sugar levels are achievable for most people through intermittent fasting, provided there are no underlying health issues that may affect these outcomes).

Relevant: Goals should be relevant to your broader objectives, ensuring they align with your values and long-term plans (Increased weight and elevated blood sugar levels are indeed my priority issues).

Time-bound: Goals should have a deadline or a specific timeframe to provide a sense of urgency and help maintain focus (I aim to lose 10 pounds and improve my blood sugar levels within the next three months using the 16/8 Method).

Managing Expectations

While intermittent fasting offers numerous health benefits, it's important to approach it with balanced expectations. Understand that changes, especially those related to weight and health markers, often occur gradually. Quick fixes are rare, and lasting improvements take time. But the slower the process is, the better the chances that results will stay.

You should be prepared for an adaptation phase where your body adjusts to new eating patterns. Temporary feelings of hunger or fatigue over a short period are normal and typically subside as your body adapts. The adaptation is over in most cases after two weeks. If you experience unwanted symptoms longer than 14 days, consider consulting the healthcare provider.

Recognize that everyone's body responds differently to intermittent fasting. Comparing your journey to others' can bring motivation and give support, but also it can lead to disappointment. Focus on your progress and how you feel and use the best tool that exists in communication - discernment. Discernment is like a filter or a prism that helps to separate needed from not needed, harmful from beneficial, and encouragement from envy.

Strategies for Achieving Goals and Tracking Process

If you have a significant long-term goal, break it down into smaller, more manageable milestones. Celebrating these smaller achievements can provide motivation and a sense of accomplishment along the way. Use printed or handmade calendars to keep a record of your achievements and draw some smileys and positive symbols along the road.

It will also help you, it you would keep track of your progress towards your goals. This could involve regular weigh-ins, tracking your fasting periods, or noting changes in how your clothes fit. Adjust your goals and strategies as needed based on your observations. As you make progress, your initial goals might no longer align with your current situation or aspirations. It's okay to reassess and set new goals that better match your evolved perspective on health and wellness. Here's how to effectively monitor your journey and make adjustments to your goals and methods.

Depending on your goals, select appropriate metrics to track your progress. If your aim is weight loss, regular weigh-ins using a scale and measurements of waist circumference can be helpful. For health improvements, you might track blood pressure, blood sugar levels, or cholesterol. But not all progress can be measured numerically. Pay attention to how you feel—energy levels, sleep quality, mental clarity, and overall wellbeing are significant indicators of the benefits of intermittent fasting.

Share your goals with friends, family, or a support group who understand and support your intermittent fasting journey. They can provide encouragement, accountability, and advice when you encounter challenges.

And also, be flexible and kind to yourself: Flexibility is key. Life events, stress, and health issues can impact your ability to stick strictly to your intermittent fasting schedule or meet your goals precisely as planned. Be willing to adjust your approach and be kind to yourself during less productive phases. Do not feel disappointed if the desired changes won't happen right away: consider giving it time or adjusting your approach/goal.

Self-acceptance, gratitude, and kindness are crucial elements in every uneasy period of our lives. You will experience joy and will be proud of yourself if your goals are achieved, but consider it ultimate importance to love and respect yourself regardless of the outcome. Imagine yourself as a loving parent who sends your child on a journey of self-discovery and trial of wrong and right. That way you will feel more secure and safe and won't punish yourself for mistakes.

Reflecting on Progress

Regular Check-ins on your goal are small steps and small steps bring more precision to a goal than a big major leap. Set a regular schedule for reviewing your progress, such as weekly or monthly. Compare your current status against your goals and the metrics you've established. Do not compare yourself with someone´s other experience, compare yourself only with yourself and your progress.

Checking your process daily might be overwhelming and not beneficial. If you wish to check your weight more often than weekly, make it at least every 3rd day. The best time to measure weight is mornings after bowel movement. Try to measure weights always in the same period of the day. For example, compare morning weight with morning weight and so on. Body weight can fluctuate greatly during the day because of body fluids, so don't be shocked in case your weight in the evening differs from that in the morning.

Celebrate small victories along the way, even if it feels as if they are meaningless. These might include fitting into a smaller clothing size, noticing improved skin health, experiencing higher energy levels, or receiving positive health markers from your doctor. Share your joyful moments with your close ones or write them down in your gratitude journal. Decide on a small treat in case of celebration: it can be anything you can imagine, from some tasty food to an item to shop. But be disciplined and true to yourself and don't search for victories in everything, making it an excuse for every treat you will allow to yourself. Find the balance between inner child and inner adult and try to hold this balance along your way to the goals.

3 NUTRITION AND DIET CONSIDERATIONS

When you start intermittent fasting, your eating habits change, therefore it becomes very important to pay attention to the composition and quality of your food at the times when you eat. This chapter explores the vital food and nutrition factors to maximize the health benefits of intermittent fasting.

Understanding the Female Body After 50

Significant physiological changes that impact hormone balance, metabolism, and general health happen to women as they enter their 50s. It's important to understand these changes to adopt dietary and lifestyle choices that promote wellbeing during this transformative period.

The Shift in Metabolism

One of the most obvious bodily changes that happen beyond 50 is a change in metabolism. The impact of this slowing on weight and health is significant. A decrease in metabolic rate is brought about by changes to cellular activity and a loss of muscle mass. This is why women may gain weight, especially around the belly, even if their diet and amount of exercise remain the same. This metabolic shift may make it harder to maintain an active lifestyle and may also have an effect on energy levels.

To balance these changes, strategies such as increasing resistance and strength training exercises might help preserve muscle mass and, thus, support a more active metabolism. Adding more nutrient-dense, high-protein, high-fiber meals to one's diet can help regulate weight and enhance overall health.

Hormonal Changes and Their Effects

Estrogen levels rise and subsequently decline throughout the menopausal phase, causing significant hormonal changes. A reduction in estrogen can result in a variety of symptoms, including mood swings, hot flashes, sleeplessness, changes in bone density, and changes in skin suppleness, as estrogen is necessary for so many bodily functions. Moreover, the reduction in estrogen is closely linked to the modifications in metabolism that are seen during this period, as estrogen controls both body weight and metabolism.

Hormonal changes can also impact energy levels, weight management, and the chance of acquiring chronic illnesses including type 2 diabetes and cardiovascular disease. These changes include adjustments in thyroid function and insulin sensitivity.

Additionally, it's critical to collaborate closely with healthcare professionals to address any health issues and create an individual strategy that supports each person's desires and requirements at this important stage of life.

Importance of Balanced Nutrition for Women Over 50

Due to significant changes in their bodies, women entering their 50s and beyond need to reevaluate their dietary needs. Balanced nutrition becomes essential for sustaining an active lifestyle, managing age-related changes, and supporting overall health. In order to address specific concerns such preserving bone density, muscular mass, and metabolic efficiency, careful evaluation of dietary habits is necessary.

Increased Protein Intake

Sarcopenia, a natural aging process marked by a loss of muscle mass, can negatively impact one's strength, flexibility, and metabolic well-being. In order to stop this loss and maintain strength and muscle mass, you must consume more protein. Foods strong in protein, such as lean meats, fish, dairy products, lentils, and tofu, not only provide the building blocks for muscle repair but also aid in satiety and weight management.

Calcium and Vitamin D

Women are more susceptible to osteoporosis as they become older, especially after menopause when their estrogen levels drop and impact bone density. Vitamin D and calcium are essential for keeping bones healthy. Vitamin D improves calcium absorption, while calcium maintains bone integrity. Good sources of calcium include dairy products, salmon, leafy green vegetables, and fortified meals. Sunlight exposure, fatty fish, and supplements—if prescribed by a medical professional—are good sources of vitamin D. Together, these nutrients maintain bone density and lower the chance of fractures.

Iron and B12

Hemoglobin, the protein in red blood cells that transports oxygen throughout the body, is made possible only by iron. To avoid anemia, women over 50—especially those who are heavily menstruating due to the changes in menopause—need to be sure they are getting enough iron in their diet. Lean meats, shellfish, nuts, beans, and fortified cereals are good sources.

Red blood cell formation, DNA synthesis, and neuron function all depend on vitamin B12. It is good to think about B12-fortified meals or supplements since the body's capacity to absorb B12 declines with age. Because animal products contain the majority of B12, supplementing is especially important for people who eat a plant-based diet.

Antioxidants and Healthy Fats

Antioxidants combat oxidative stress and inflammation, which are linked to aging and chronic diseases. A diet rich in fruits, vegetables, nuts, and seeds provides a variety of antioxidants that promote health and longevity.

Healthy fats, especially omega-3 fatty acids, are vital for heart health, cognitive function, and joint mobility. Sources include fatty fish, flaxseeds, chia seeds, walnuts, and avocados. These fats support hormone production, which is particularly important as estrogen levels decline.

Below is a list of important supplements, vitamins, and electrolytes, including their general recommended daily allowance (RDA) for the average adult and the adjusted norms for women over 50.

	Average Adult	Women over 50	Needs and Benefits
Calcium	1000mg	1200g	Crucial for maintaining bone health and reducing the risk of osteoporosis, is beneficial for sleep.
Vitamin D	600-800 IU	800-1000 IU	Helps in calcium absorption and is vital for bone, muscle, and immune health.
Vitamin B12	2,4 mcg	2,4 mcg	The need for Vitamin B12 remains consistent, but women over 50 are advised to get it from fortified foods or supplements due to the increased risk of malabsorption.

Magnesium	Men: 400-420 mg; Women: 310-320 mg	320 mg	Magnesium supports bone health, muscle function, and over 300 enzyme reactions. Helps to establish a healthy night´s sleep.
Omega-3 Fatty Acid	1,1-1,6 g	No specific increase	Vital for heart health and cognitive function, suggesting a focus on adequate intake or supplementation.
Vitamin B6	1,3 mg	1,5 mg	Important for cognitive health and immune function.
Iron	Women before menopause: 18 mg	8 mg in menopause, but higher if heavy bleedings still occur	Producing hemoglobin and supporting overall energy levels and immune function.
Fiber	25-30 g	21 g	For digestive health and maintaining healthy blood sugar levels. The recommended intake slightly decreases due to possible lower calorie needs.
Potassium	2600 – 3400 mg	2600 mg	Vital for heart health, muscle function, and blood pressure regulation. The need remains substantial to counteract hypertension risk and maintain cellular function.
Zinc	Men: 11 mg; Women: 8	8 mg	Supports immune function, wound healing, and DNA synthesis. While the recommended

	mg		intake doesn't increase, maintaining adequate levels is crucial for overall health and disease prevention.
Vitamin C	75 mg	75 mg	Crucial for the immune system, skin health, and collagen production. It also plays a significant role in wound healing and as an antioxidant, protecting cells from damage.
Vitamin E	15 mg	15 mg	Serves as a powerful antioxidant that protects cells from oxidative stress, which is particularly beneficial for aging skin and immune health. Supports eye health and cardiovascular function.
Vitamin A	700 mcg	700 mcg	Maintains healthy vision, skin, and immune function. It also plays a critical role in cell growth and differentiation.
Folate (Folic Acid)	400 mcg	400 mcg	Helps the production of red blood cells and prevents anemia. Supports cardiovascular health.
Coenzyme Q 10	Commonly 30-200 mg	Commonly 30-200 mg	A powerful antioxidant, helps generate energy in cells and is thought to enhance heart health and blood sugar regulation. Regenerates cells from

			damage like viruses.
Sodium	Less than 2300 mg	Less than 1500 mg	Essential for fluid balance, nerve transmission, and muscle function, plays a big role in hypertension and cardiovascular diseases
Iodine	150 mcg	150 mcg, depending on the thyroid condition	Production of thyroid hormones, which regulate metabolism, growth, and development. Proper thyroid function is important for energy levels, maintaining a healthy weight, and preventing conditions like hypothyroidism.

In the table below you will find information about foods that are rich in some of those minerals and vitamins. Note that it is very difficult to cover the daily needs just by food intake and consider purchasing the supplements for at least a short time, for example, 90-120 days.

Calcium	Dairy products: milk (especially goat), yogurt, cheese Leafy green vegetables: kale, collard greens, broccoli Fortified foods: orange juice, plant-based milk Fish with bones: canned salmon, sardines Almonds
Vitamin D	Fatty fish: salmon, mackerel, tuna Egg yolks Fortified foods: milk, orange juice, cereals Mushrooms exposed to sunlight Cod liver oil
Vitamin B12	Animal products: meat, fish, poultry, eggs Dairy products: milk, cheese, yogurt Nutritional yeast Fortified plant-based milk

Magnesium	Nuts and seeds: almonds, pumpkin seeds, chia seeds Whole grains: brown rice, quinoa, whole wheat Leafy green vegetables: spinach, Swiss chard Legumes: black beans, lentils Avocado
Omega-3 Fatty Acid	Fatty fish: salmon, mackerel, sardines Walnuts Flaxseeds and flaxseed oil Chia seeds Hemp seeds Canola oil
Vitamin B6	Poultry: chicken, turkey Fish: salmon, tuna Potatoes and other starchy vegetables Non-citrus fruits: bananas, avocados
Iron	Red meat: beef, lamb Poultry: turkey, chicken Seafood: oysters, clams, tuna Legumes: lentils, chickpeas Spinach and other leafy greens Nettle tea
Fiber	Legumes: beans, lentils, chickpeas Berries: raspberries, blackberries Whole grains: oats, barley, bran Nuts and seeds: almonds, chia seeds, flaxseeds Vegetables: artichokes, broccoli
Potassium	Fruits: bananas, oranges, cantaloupe Vegetables: spinach, sweet potatoes, tomatoes Beans: white beans, kidney beans Potatoes: white and sweet potatoes Dairy products: yogurt, milk
Zinc	Meat: beef, lamb, pork Shellfish: oysters, crab, lobster Legumes: chickpeas, lentils, beans Nuts and seeds: pumpkin seeds, cashews Dairy products: milk, cheese
Vitamin C	Citrus fruits such as oranges, grapefruits, and lemons Strawberries, raspberries, and blueberries Kiwi fruit Bell peppers (red, green, yellow) Dark leafy greens like spinach and kale

	Tomatoes and tomato juice Broccoli and Brussels sprouts
Vitamin E	Nuts and seeds, such as almonds, sunflower seeds, and hazelnuts Spinach and other green leafy vegetables Vegetable oils like sunflower, safflower, and wheat germ oil Avocados Shellfish Pumpkins and sweet potatoes
Vitamin A	Liver and fish oils Sweet potatoes, carrots, and squash Green leafy vegetables like kale, spinach, and collard greens Bell peppers Cantaloupe and apricots Dairy products like milk and cheese
Folate (Folic Acid)	Dark green leafy vegetables such as spinach and mustard greens Asparagus and Brussels sprouts Legumes like beans, peas, and lentils Nuts and seeds Beef liver Poultry, pork, and shellfish Whole grains
Coenzyme Q 10	(Best to use as a supplement). Organ meats such as liver and kidney Beef, pork, and chicken Fatty fish like trout, herring, and mackerel Spinach, broccoli, and cauliflower Soybeans, lentils, and peanuts Oranges and strawberries
Iodine	Seaweed, such as kelp, nori, and wakame Dairy products like milk, cheese, and yogurt Iodized table salt Fish and shellfish Eggs Prunes

Let's Talk About Calcium, Again

As was already noted, the increased risk of osteoporosis and bone density loss that comes with aging and menopause makes it vital to consume enough calcium. For women over 50, the recommended daily intake (RDA) for calcium is 1,200 mg daily. This is more than what is advised for younger folks, highlighting the necessity of consuming more calcium to support the maintenance of strong and healthy bones. It essential that they consume foods high in calcium, such as dairy products, fortified plant-based milks, leafy green vegetables, and fish in cans with bones, in order to achieve these requirements. In addition, it's critical to consume enough vitamin D to enhance the body's ability to absorb and use calcium.

If you choose to use calcium supplements, calcium fructoborate is something I wholeheartedly suggest. A naturally occurring substance that contains calcium, boron, and fructose is called calcium fructoborate. It is mostly present in vegetables, fruits, and some types of legumes. Because of its distinct molecular structure, this substance is highly bioavailable—that is, the body can readily absorb and use it—which makes it especially intriguing. Its advantages include impacts on bone and joint health, hormone balance, and anti-inflammatory and antioxidative properties as a mineral.

Of course, if there is a significant deficiency of calcium in the diet, supplementing with capsules and powders is insufficient. The best strategy to maintain healthy calcium levels is to take mineral supplements along with foods high in calcium. The approximate calcium content (per 100g) of the following foods is listed:

Cow milk	120 mg
Goat milk	320 mg
Cow milk yogurts	120 mg, depending on yogurt
Cheese	Up to 1100 mg, depending on cheese
Kale	150 mg
Collard Greens	230 mg
Spinach	120 mg
Broccoli	60 mg
Plant-based milk	120 mg, depending on product and plant

ned salmon with bones	200 mg
...uines with bones	380 mg
Almonds and almond butter	250 mg / 55 mg
Tofu	175 mg
Bok Choy	150 mg
Dried figs	140 mg
Sesame seeds and tahini	780 mg / 250 mg
Poppy seeds	1400 mg
White beans	240 mg
Chickpeas	50 mg
Black-eyed peas	40 mg
Butternut squash	50 mg
Sweet potatoes	80 mg
Seaweed	55 mg
Chia seeds	630 mg

The Potential of Urolithin A for Women Over 50

Urolithin A is a transformative compound produced by gut bacteria when they metabolize ellagitannins, substances found in foods like pomegranates, berries, nuts, and red wine. This compound has sparked considerable interest due to its potential benefits for mitochondrial health and cellular longevity, which are particularly relevant for women over 50 dealing with aging cells and declining mitochondrial efficiency.

Urolithin A promotes mitophagy, the selective recycling of damaged mitochondria and the research suggests that Urolithin A can improve muscle strength and endurance by boosting mitochondrial function. This benefit helps maintain mobility, reduce physical fatigue, and enhance overall physical performance.

Some preliminary studies indicate that Urolithin A may also support brain health and cognitive function, providing potential protection against neurodegenerative diseases like Alzheimer's, which are of particular concern in aging populations. It has also significant anti-inflammatory and antioxidant effects that help mitigate chronic inflammation and oxidative stress, both of which contribute to chronic diseases and the aging process.

Dietary Sources of Urolithin A

Currently, Urolithin A itself is not available as a dietary supplement. However, you can encourage its natural production by consuming foods rich in ellagitannins. Including pomegranates, strawberries, raspberries, walnuts, and oak-aged red wines in your diet may promote the gut microbiota's natural synthesis of Urolithin A.

What to Eat During the Eating Window?

The eating window is an essential period for those who follow intermittent fasting. The success and health advantages of your fasting journey depend not only on when you eat, but also on what you eat. Healthy metabolism, increased energy levels, and ensuring your body gets the vital nutrients it needs to flourish may all be achieved with nutrient-dense, well-balanced meals. Naturally, your meals must align with the intermittent fasting strategy you have selected. For instance, if your eating window is eight hours, attempt to fit in no more than three meals. The ideal time between meals is three to four hours, with each meal lasting no more than an hour.

Your eating window is longer if you selected the 12/12 Method, but you should still aim to plan three meals and extend the time between them to six or seven hours. Any amount of calories consumed, even during a short snack period, counts as one meal. To avoid cravings for snacks in between meals, I suggest eating during meal times well to feel satisfied.

The meal preparation would be more challenging if you went with the OMAD Method. It takes extensive understanding of your organism's requirements to do this. To keep your body healthy and energized without falling into survival mode, you must consume as many nutrients in one meal as you can.

The following general suggestions can help you maximize your eating window:

Prioritize Protein

Sustaining muscle mass, mending tissues, and regulating blood sugar levels all depend on high-quality protein sources during the meal window. A range of protein sources should be included, especially dairy and eggs for people who consume animal products, lean meats (such as chicken, turkey, and lean cuts of beef), fish and shellfish (such as shrimp, mackerel, salmon, and sardines), and plant-based proteins (such as lentils, beans, chickpeas, tofu, and tempeh).

In addition to promoting physical health, proteins also help with satiety, which can help control appetite during fasting times.

Incorporate Whole Grains

Whole grains offer essential vitamins, minerals, fiber, and slow-digesting carbohydrates that provide sustained energy. Options like quinoa, brown rice, barley, and whole wheat are excellent choices. They support digestive health and maintain steady blood sugar levels.

Moderate Fruits and lots of Vegetables

Fruits and vegetables are rich in vitamins, minerals, antioxidants, and fiber. Aim for a variety of colors to ensure a wide range of nutrients. These foods can help reduce inflammation, support immune function, and contribute to overall health. Leafy greens, berries, cruciferous vegetables (like broccoli and Brussels sprouts), and orange vegetables (like carrots and sweet potatoes) are particularly beneficial. But be careful with high fruit intake: if your goal is to lose weight, reducing fruit intake might be a big help, due to the fructose (easy sugar) absorbed in the digestive tract. Also, try to eat fruits as an independent meal or before your real meal, for better digestion.

Choose Healthy Fats

Absorption of fat-soluble vitamins (A, D, E, and K) and hormone production both depend on healthy fats. Add sources of monounsaturated and polyunsaturated fats, such as omega-3-rich fatty fish, avocados, nuts, and seeds (almonds, walnuts, flaxseeds, and chia seeds). These fats can aid in the management of inflammation and support cardiovascular health. Selecting healthy fats with the optimal Omega-3 to Omega-6 ratio is particularly crucial. The body needs both of those fatty acids to function, however Omega-6 is more quickly absorbed and bound by enzymes than Omega-3.

Flaxseed, chia seed, walnut, and hemp seed oils are some of the finest for increasing your consumption of omega-3 fatty acids relative to omega-6 when it comes to cooking and salad dressing. It's important to remember that several of these oils—flaxseed and chia seed oil, in particular—have low smoke points and shouldn't be used for cooking at high temperatures. To preserve their nutritional value, they are best added to cooked dishes or used in dressings. Compared to most typical cooking oils like corn or sunflower oil, canola oil has a better fatty acid profile and is heat-stable for regular cooking.

What about dessert?

During your eating window, it is allowed to eat desserts, if it doesn't disturb your diet goal. For example, if your blood sugar levels are too high and you need to lose weight, healthy desserts like chia pudding or low-sugar chocolate mousse could be absolutely fine. If you allow yourself to eat bakery and more sweet stuff, it should not influence your intermittent fasting process, and should be consumed only if your goals allow it.

Focus on Fiber

Fiber plays a crucial role in digestive health, blood sugar regulation, and cholesterol management. Sources of high-quality fiber include vegetables, fruits, whole grains, and legumes. Some of the best fiber-rich products are chia seeds, flaxseed, and psyllium husk. The best way is to prepare them like pudding in water or milk (also plant-based milk) and let them swell and thicken. Important information about fiber-rich nutrition is that the need for fluid increases. In case there is not enough fluid in the body, fiber can cause constipation.

Stay Hydrated

While hydration should be maintained throughout the day, including during fasting periods, the eating window is a good time to include hydrating foods and beverages that contribute to your overall fluid intake.

The Importance of Hydration During Intermittent Fasting

Staying hydrated is essential for the effectiveness and health benefits of intermittent fasting, especially while the body adjusts to new eating habits. The body uses water to carry out various functions, including digestion, absorption of nutrients, and elimination of toxins. It also helps to maintain energy levels, mental clarity, and physical performance—all of which are especially important when fasting.

Why Hydration Matters

During periods of fasting, the body continues to lose water due to normal physiological processes like respiration, sweating, and cellular metabolism. When we don't eat frequently, which typically increases our daily fluid consumption, the risk of dehydration increases. In addition to having a decreased thirst response, with growing age we should drink more water since we are adjusting to changes in hormone levels and metabolism that could affect fluid balance.

Effects of Dehydration

Dehydration can lead to a range of symptoms that not only affect wellbeing but can also hinder the effectiveness of the intermittent fasting regimen. These include:

Fatigue and Lethargy: Dehydration can lead to feelings of tiredness, affecting energy levels and motivation.

Headaches and Dizziness: Common symptoms of dehydration, impacting daily activities and overall quality of life.

Impaired Cognitive Function: Concentration, memory, and alertness can suffer, making it harder to focus and be productive.

Elimination: Adequate hydration is essential for digestive health, particularly in preventing constipation. It is also needed due to increased sweating for those experiencing hot and cold flashes. Dehydration is often noticeable through urination: urine becomes more cark in color and may have a strong smell. Also, amounts of urine can change and become less. Strongly concentrated urine may lead to urine tract infections due to a lack of natural cleansing.

Hunger Misinterpretation: Thirst can often be mistaken for hunger, leading to challenges in adhering to fasting periods. Craving for something sweet is one of the symptoms of dehydration.

Dry Skin and Lips/Mouth: Those are direct symptoms of the body craving more water in long term. Notice how your skin and lips get better, when you start to drink more water.

Hydration Strategies for Intermittent Fasting

To ensure adequate hydration during intermittent fasting, consider incorporating a variety of fluids that count towards your daily intake:

Water: The most straightforward and effective way to stay hydrated. Aim for at least 8-10 glasses (about 2-2.5 liters) per day, adjusting based on your activity level, climate, and personal needs. The best formula to calculate your daily need is between half an ounce and an ounce of water for each pound of body weight (or 30ml per kg). There are many water intake calculators that you can find on the internet, in case you want to be sure. Starting a day with a glass of lukewarm water (or even more warm) can help your gall bladder to become active and promote detoxification.

I do not recommend drinking water with your meal: it can dilute the stomach acid and make food digestion difficult. As a result, problems like bloating or heartburn can occur. What is more beneficial, is to drink your water during the day, 10-15 minutes before meal intake, or to add lemon or lime to make it sourer and support digestion. Otherwise, juices and herbal teas are perfect alternatives for your drinks during meal intake.

Electrolyte-infused Water: Adding electrolytes can help maintain the body's balance of minerals, especially important during longer fasting periods or for those who engage in regular physical activity.

Herbal Teas: Non-caffeinated herbal teas are a great way to increase fluid intake while offering a soothing, flavorful beverage option. They can also provide therapeutic benefits, such as chamomile for relaxation or peppermint for digestion. Notice that black tea and green tea could lead to more fluid elimination, so it is not recommended to use those teas to soothe your thirst.

Bone Broth: For those practicing less strict forms of intermittent fasting, bone broth can provide hydration along with essential nutrients like minerals and amino acids.

Fruit and Vegetable Juices: In moderation and as part of the eating window, fresh, low-sodium vegetable juices or diluted fruit juices can contribute to hydration and nutrient intake. Diluted juices can be an even better choice, in case weight loss is one of your goals or you suffer from elevated blood sugar levels or liver issues. Take 1/3 of juice and dilute it with 2/3 of water.

It's important to listen to your body and drink fluids throughout the day, not just during your eating window. Your daily fluid intake can depend on weather and physical activity, and sometimes even on the menu. If you forget to drink, keep a bottle somewhere nearby as a reminder. You can connect water intake with the periods, for example, finishing one bottle until 3 PM, or even use hydration apps that remind you to drink a cup of water.

Bulletproof Coffee and Coffee/Tea with Butter

There are opinions, that Bulletproof coffee and tea are essential drinks to have during intermittent fasting. If you find it interesting, you can find the information you need on the Internet. The founder of Biohacking Dave Asprey came up with this term and speaks often of its benefits for the body. It's a blend of coffee, grass-fed unsalted butter, and medium-chain triglyceride (MCT) oil. This high-fat beverage has gained popularity within ketogenic diet circles and among those practicing intermittent fasting for its purported benefits, including enhanced energy, increased satiety, and improved mental clarity. Similarly, adding butter to tea, especially in variations like Tibetan tea, shares a tradition of incorporating high-fat elements to sustain energy and warmth.

The Composition and Benefits

Coffee/Tea: Both serve as the beverage base, providing caffeine, which is known for its stimulant properties, enhancing alertness and concentration.

Grass-fed Butter: Rich in omega-3 fatty acids, butyrate, and vitamins A, D, E, and K2. Grass-fed butter is preferred for its higher nutritional quality over regular butter.

MCT Oil: Extracted primarily from coconut oil, MCT oil contains fats that are metabolized differently from other types of fats. They're quickly absorbed and converted into ketone bodies, providing a rapid energy source and potentially aiding in ketosis for those on a ketogenic diet.

Purported Benefits

Caffeine and good fats work together to deliver energy gradually, preventing the crash that comes with most typical high-carb breakfasts. Because of its high fat content, it promotes satiety and might intensify sensations of fullness, hence decreasing appetite and possibly calorie consumption overall. Certain sources mention enhanced mental clarity and focus, which they partly credit to the effects of MCT oil's ketone bodies and caffeine. Bulletproof coffee can complement a ketogenic lifestyle and help maintain ketosis. It is supposed to promote ketogenic diets by offering a high-fat, low-carb choice.

Considerations and Criticisms

Bulletproof coffee has its opposing viewpoints, even if it can work with some diet plans. Bulletproof coffee lacks important components present in entire foods, like fiber, protein, and numerous vitamins and minerals, therefore consuming it as a meal replacement could result in nutritional deficits. Furthermore, because it is high in calories, consuming it in addition to a regular diet without taking total calorie intake into account could lead to weight gain. Additionally, there are certain heart health issues. The saturated fat level of butter and MCT oil raises worries about possible effects on heart health, while the evidence is conflicting and may vary depending on the individual and diet composition.

Meal Planning for Success

Preparing meals carefully is the first step towards a successful intermittent fasting journey, especially for individuals who may need to take certain nutritional factors into account. A well-thought-out meal plan ensures that you will maintain your energy levels, reach your health goals, and maximize the nutrients you consume during your eating windows. These practical meal planning ideas can help you minimize stress, streamline the process, and get the most out of your intermittent fasting program.

Plan Your Eating Window

Establish the format of your eating window based on your fasting method and lifestyle. Choose how many meals and snacks you want to have during your eating period, regardless of whether you're using a 16/8, 5:2, or other intermittent fasting approach. This will assist you in determining the right amount and variety of meals to consume to meet your nutritional requirements without overeating.

Create a Flexible Meal Template

Create a customizable meal plan that incorporates a range of dietary groups. For instance, try to have a supply of protein, good fat, a variety of vegetables, and a mix of carbohydrates with every meal. By using this form, you can guarantee balanced nutrition and simplify the meal planning process.

Batch Cooking and Meal Prep

Prepare meals or meal components in advance to save time and ensure you have healthy options readily available. Cooking in advance reduces meal preparation time and it is very convenient for busy women. However, if you have the opportunity to cook every day fresh, it could be beneficial to the whole process. Eating food that is prepared days before may increase histamine levels and have an impact on your liver health.

Keep Healthy Snacks on Hand

During your eating window, it's helpful to have healthy snacks readily available, especially if your eating window is longer. Options like Greek yogurt, nuts, seeds, sliced vegetables with hummus, or a piece of fruit can provide a nutritious boost without requiring extensive preparation time.

Stay Flexible and Listen to Your Body

While it's beneficial to have a plan, it's equally important to remain flexible and attuned to your body's signals. Appetite and energy levels can fluctuate, especially as you adjust to an intermittent fasting schedule. Be prepared to adjust portion sizes and meal composition as needed to satisfy hunger and support your body's needs.

Review and Adjust Regularly

Periodically review your meal plan's effectiveness in meeting your health and wellness goals. As you progress with intermittent fasting and potentially experience changes in health, weight, or activity level, your dietary needs may also change. Be open to adjusting your meal planning strategy to continue supporting your health and fasting goals effectively.

4 IDEAS FOR MEALS AND RECIPES

At this point, you have probably chosen the method of intermittent fasting that you want to start with. In the following chapter, you will find ideas for meals according to some methods and delicious recipes to try during your intermittent fasting journey.

Recipes for OMAD Method

The best way to consume your minimum daily calories with the OMAD Method would be to extend your meal intake time to about one hour or even one hour and a half. Don´t rush and take it slow, eat a small starter, continue with the full meal, and finish with a tasty dessert. Of course, adjust according to your individual needs and preferences. All recipes are calculated per one portion.

Starters

Recipe 1: Grilled Vegetable and Hummus Platter

Ingredients:

1/2 zucchini, sliced lengthwise

1/2 bell pepper, cut into strips

5 cherry tomatoes

1/4 eggplant, sliced

1/4 cup hummus

1 tbsp olive oil

Salt and pepper to taste

Nutritional Value & Calories:

Calories: Approximately 300

Protein: 6g

Fat: 20g

Carbohydrates: 27g

Fiber: 9g

This dish is rich in fiber and provides a good dose of vitamins A and C.

Instructions:

1.   Preheat the grill or a grill pan.

2.   Brush the zucchini, bell pepper, cherry tomatoes, and eggplant slices with olive oil and season with salt and pepper.

3.   Grill the vegetables until tender and nicely charred, about 3-4 minutes per side.

4.   Arrange the grilled vegetables on a plate and serve with a side of hummus for dipping.

Recipe 2: Shrimp and Avocado Salad

Ingredients:

4 oz cooked shrimp

1/2 ripe avocado, diced

1/2 cup mixed greens

1/4 cup cherry tomatoes, halved

1 tbsp lime juice

1 tsp olive oil

Salt and pepper to taste

A pinch of chili flakes (optional)

Nutritional Value & Calories:

Calories: Approximately 300

Protein: 24g

Fat: 18g

Carbohydrates: 8g

Fiber: 5g

This salad is a great source of protein and healthy fats, particularly omega-3 fatty acids from the shrimp.

Instructions:

1. In a mixing bowl, combine the cooked shrimp, diced avocado, mixed greens, and cherry tomatoes.

2. Dress the salad with lime juice, olive oil, salt, pepper, and chili flakes if using.

3. Toss gently to combine and serve immediately.

Recipe 3: Caprese Skewers with Balsamic Glaze

Ingredients:

Nutritional Value & Calories:

4 cherry tomatoes

4 small balls of fresh mozzarella cheese

4 fresh basil leaves

2 tbsp balsamic glaze

1 tsp olive oil

Salt and pepper to taste

Calories: Approximately 300

Protein: 18g

Fat: 20g

Carbohydrates: 10g

Fiber: 1g

This starter is a good source of calcium from the mozzarella and provides a satisfying combination of flavors and textures.

Instructions:

1.   Skewer a cherry tomato, a basil leaf, and a mozzarella ball onto small skewers or cocktail sticks. Repeat for all skewers.

2.   Drizzle with olive oil and season with salt and pepper.

3.   Just before serving, drizzle with balsamic glaze for added flavor.

Main Dish

Recipe 1: Salmon Quinoa Bowl

Ingredients:

Nutritional Value & Calories:

6 oz grilled salmon

1 cup cooked quinoa

1 cup steamed broccoli

1/2 avocado, sliced

1/2 cup cherry tomatoes, halved

2 tbsp feta cheese, crumbled

Dressing: 1 tbsp olive oil, 2 tsp lemon juice, salt, and pepper to taste

Calories: Approximately 850

Protein: 45g

Fat: 50g (healthy fats from salmon, avocado, and olive oil)

Carbohydrates: 55g

Fiber: 12g

Rich in Omega-3 fatty acids, Vitamin C, Calcium, and Iron.

Instructions:

1.   Layer the cooked quinoa as a base in a large bowl.

2.   Arrange the grilled salmon, steamed broccoli, sliced avocado, and cherry tomatoes over the quinoa.

3.   Sprinkle crumbled feta cheese on top.

4.   Whisk together olive oil, lemon juice, salt, and pepper, and drizzle over the bowl.

Recipe 2: Mediterranean Chicken and Vegetable Platter

Ingredients:

8 oz roasted chicken breast

1 cup whole grain couscous, cooked

1/2 cup hummus

1 cup grilled vegetables (zucchini, bell peppers, and eggplant)

1/2 cup olives

2 tbsp almonds, chopped

Fresh herbs (parsley or cilantro), for garnish

Nutritional Value & Calories:

Calories: Approximately 900

Protein: 60g

Fat: 40g

Carbohydrates: 65g

Fiber: 14g

Rich in Vitamins A, C, E, B vitamins, and healthy fats.

Instructions:

1. Arrange cooked couscous on one side of a large plate.

2. Place roasted chicken breast alongside couscous.

3. Add a scoop of hummus and spread out grilled vegetables.

4. Scatter olives and chopped almonds over the entire plate.

5. Garnish with fresh herbs.

Recipe 3: Beef Stir-Fry with Mixed Vegetables and Brown Rice

Ingredients:

6 oz lean beef strips

2 cups mixed vegetables (carrots, broccoli, bell pepper)

1 cup brown rice, cooked

2 tbsp soy sauce (low sodium)

1 tbsp sesame oil

1 garlic clove, minced

1 tsp ginger, grated

1 tbsp sesame seeds

Nutritional Value & Calories:

Calories: Approximately 750

Protein: 45g

Fat: 25g

Carbohydrates: 80g

Fiber: 8g

Rich in Iron, Vitamin A, Vitamin C, and complex carbohydrates.

Instructions:

1.   Heat sesame oil in a wok or large skillet over medium-high heat.

2.   Add garlic and ginger, sauté for 1 minute.

3.   Add beef strips, stir-fry until browned.

4.   Add vegetables and soy sauce, continue to stir-fry until vegetables are just tender.

5.   Serve the stir-fry over a bed of brown rice, sprinkle with sesame seeds.

Deserts

Recipe 1: Berry Yogurt Parfait

Ingredients:

1 cup Greek yogurt (plain, non-fat)

1 cup mixed berries (strawberries, blueberries, raspberries)

2 tbsp honey

1/4 cup granola

Nutritional Value & Calories:

Calories: Approximately 350

Protein: 20g

Fat: 5g

Carbohydrates: 60g

Fiber: 4g

This parfait is rich in protein and antioxidants, with the berries providing a good source of vitamins.

Instructions:

1. In a glass or bowl, layer half the Greek yogurt.

2. Add a layer of mixed berries.

3. Drizzle 1 tbsp of honey over the berries.

4. Add another layer of Greek yogurt, followed by the remaining berries and honey.

5. Top with granola for crunch.

Recipe 2: Chocolate Avocado Mousse

Ingredients:	**Nutritional Value & Calories:**
1 ripe avocado	Calories: Approximately 400
1/4 cup cocoa powder	Protein: 6g
1/4 cup coconut milk	Fat: 24g
2 tbsp maple syrup	Carbohydrates: 45g
1 tsp vanilla extract	Fiber: 12g
A pinch of salt	This dessert offers healthy fats and fiber, making it both filling and indulgent.

Instructions:

1.   Blend the ripe avocado, cocoa powder, coconut milk, maple syrup, vanilla extract, and a pinch of salt in a food processor until smooth.

2.   Chill the mixture in the refrigerator for at least an hour.

3.   Serve cold, garnished with a few berries or a sprinkle of shredded coconut if desired.

Recipe 3: Baked Apple with Cinnamon and Nuts

Ingredients:	Nutritional Value & Calories:
1 large apple, cored	Calories: Approximately 300
2 tbsp chopped walnuts	Protein: 3g
1 tbsp honey	Fat: 10g
1/2 tsp ground cinnamon	Carbohydrates: 53g
1/4 tsp nutmeg	Fiber: 6g
A splash of lemon juice	This warm, comforting dessert is low in fat and high in fiber, with cinnamon providing anti-inflammatory benefits.

Instructions:

1. Preheat the oven to 350°F (175°C).

2. Place the cored apple on a baking sheet.

3. Mix the chopped walnuts, honey, cinnamon, nutmeg, and lemon juice in a small bowl.

4. Stuff this mixture into the center of the apple.

5. Bake in the preheated oven for about 20-25 minutes, or until the apple is tender.

6. Serve warm, possibly with a dollop of low-fat vanilla yogurt.

Recipes for 16/8 Method

Skipping Dinner

For a woman following the 16:8 intermittent fasting method and skipping dinner, breakfast becomes a crucial meal that needs to be nutrient-dense to sustain energy throughout the day and until the next morning. Here are some breakfast and lunch examples designed to pack in essential nutrients, including a good dose of calcium, to support overall health.

Breakfast 1: Protein-Packed Green Smoothie

Ingredients:

Nutritional Value & Calories:

1 cup fortified plant-based milk (almond, soy, or oat milk)

½ cup Greek yogurt

1 cup fresh kale leaves (stemmed and chopped)

½ banana

2 tablespoons chia seeds

A handful of almonds or 1 tablespoon almond butter

Ice cubes (optional, for texture)

Calories: Approximately 441

Protein: 27.1g

Fat: 21.7g

Carbohydrates: 42g

Fiber: 15.3g

This green smoothie provides a refreshing and energizing start to the day, with the kale and fortified plant-based milk offering a substantial calcium boost.

Instructions:

Blend all ingredients until smooth.

Breakfast 2: Savory Oatmeal with Kale and Poached Egg

Ingredients:

½ cup rolled oats cooked in fortified plant-based milk

1 cup chopped kale (sautéed lightly)

1 poached egg

1 tablespoon grated Parmesan cheese

Salt, pepper, and a drizzle of olive oil for seasoning

Nutritional Value & Calories:

Calories: Approximately 317

Protein: 17.2g

Fat: 14.3g

Carbohydrates: 33.6g

Fiber: 5.3g

This hearty meal combines the benefits of fiber-rich oats, nutrient-dense kale, and the protein from the egg, with an added calcium kick from the cheese.

Instructions:

1. Prepare the oatmeal as per usual but use fortified plant-based milk instead of water.

2. Stir in the sautéed kale, and top with a poached egg and grated Parmesan.

3. Season with salt, pepper, and a drizzle of olive oil.

Breakfast 3: Yogurt Parfait with Mixed Berries and Nuts

Ingredients:

Nutritional Value & Calories:

1 cup Greek yogurt

Calories: Approximately 405

½ cup mixed berries

Protein: 29.7g

¼ cup granola

Fat: 12.2g

A sprinkle of chia seeds and sliced almonds

Carbohydrates: 49.2g

Fiber: 8.7g

A drizzle of honey or maple syrup for sweetness (optional)

This parfait is not only visually appealing but packed with calcium from the yogurt and almonds, antioxidants from the berries, and omega-3 fatty acids from the chia seeds.

Instructions:

1. Layer the Greek yogurt with mixed berries and granola in a bowl or glass.

2. Top with chia seeds, sliced almonds, and a drizzle of honey or maple syrup if desired.

Lunch 1: Quinoa and Roasted Vegetable Salad

Ingredients:

Nutritional Value & Calories:

1 cup cooked quinoa

2 cups mixed vegetables (broccoli, bell peppers, and cherry tomatoes) roasted

¼ cup feta cheese, crumbled

A handful of pumpkin seeds

Dressing: Olive oil, lemon juice, salt, and pepper to taste

Calories: Approximately 680

Protein: 23g

Fat: 37.6g

Carbohydrates: 65.2g

Fiber: 12g

This salad combines high-fiber quinoa and vegetables with the calcium-rich feta cheese, making it a balanced and filling lunch option.

Instructions:

1. Toss the cooked quinoa with the roasted vegetables.

2. Top with crumbled feta cheese and pumpkin seeds.

3. Drizzle with a simple dressing of olive oil, lemon juice, salt, and pepper.

Lunch 2: Spinach and Mushroom Omelet with Avocado

Ingredients:

2 large eggs

1 cup fresh spinach

½ cup sliced mushrooms

¼ avocado, sliced

1 tablespoon grated Parmesan cheese

Salt, pepper, and herbs to taste

Nutritional Value & Calories:

Calories: Approximately 261

Protein: 16.9g

Fat: 19.2g

Carbohydrates: 8g

Fiber: 4.4g

This omelet packs a punch with protein from the eggs, calcium from the spinach and cheese, and healthy fats from the avocado.

Instructions:

1. Whisk the eggs and pour them into a hot, greased pan.

2. Add the spinach and mushrooms to one side of the omelet as it cooks.

3. Once set, sprinkle with Parmesan, fold over, and serve with sliced avocado on the side.

Lunch 3: Lentil Soup with Kale and Almonds

Ingredients:

1 cup lentils (cooked according to package instructions, rich in protein and fiber)

2 cups vegetable broth

1 cup chopped kale

¼ cup sliced almonds

Seasonings: garlic, onion, cumin, salt, and pepper to taste

A squeeze of lemon juice for brightness

Nutritional Value & Calories:

Calories: Approximately 463

Protein: 28.9g

Fat: 15.9g

Carbohydrates: 60g

Fiber: 20.8g

This hearty soup offers a comforting meal that's high in protein, fiber, and calcium, thanks to the lentils, kale, and almonds.

Instruction:

1. In a large pot, sauté garlic and onion until translucent.

2. Add cooked lentils and vegetable broth, bringing to a simmer.

3. Stir in chopped kale and seasonings, cooking until the kale is wilted.

4. Serve hot, topped with sliced almonds and a squeeze of lemon juice.

Skipping breakfast

When adopting the 16:8 intermittent fasting method with breakfast skipped but dinner included, your lunch serves as the important first meal of the day. It should be both satisfying and nutrient-rich, setting a strong nutritional foundation for the rest of your eating window.

Lunch 1: Salmon and Avocado Salad

Ingredients:

Nutritional Value & Calories:

4 oz grilled salmon

2 cups mixed greens (like spinach and arugula)

½ ripe avocado, sliced

¼ cup sliced strawberries

2 tablespoons chopped walnuts

Dressing: A mix of olive oil, balsamic vinegar, mustard, salt, and pepper

Calories: Approximately 613

Protein: 31.8g

Fat: 48.5g

Carbohydrates: 22.7g

Fiber: 9g

This meal combines heart-healthy fats, lean protein, and a variety of vitamins and minerals, providing a balanced and refreshing start to your eating period.

Instructions:

1. On a large plate, arrange the mixed greens and top with grilled salmon, sliced avocado, strawberries, and chopped walnuts.

2. Whisk together the dressing ingredients and drizzle over the salad.

Lunch 2: Chickpea and Sweet Potato Bowl

Ingredients:

Nutritional Value & Calories:

Ingredients:	Nutritional Value & Calories:
1 cup roasted sweet potato cubes	Calories: Approximately 667
½ cup cooked chickpeas	Protein: 23.3g
1 cup steamed broccoli florets	Fat: 28.5g
¼ cup crumbled feta cheese	Carbohydrates: 85.4g
2 tablespoons tahini sauce	Fiber: 21.4g
A sprinkle of sesame seeds and a squeeze of lemon juice for garnish	This bowl is not only hearty and satisfying but also packed with nutrients essential for bone health and energy maintenance.

Instructions:

1. In a medium bowl, combine the roasted sweet potato cubes, cooked chickpeas, and steamed broccoli.

2. Top with crumbled feta cheese and drizzle with tahini sauce.

3. Garnish with sesame seeds and a squeeze of fresh lemon juice.

Lunch 3: Lentil Soup with Kale

Ingredients:	Nutritional Value & Calories:
1 cup cooked lentils	Calories: Approximately 350
2 cups vegetable broth	Protein: 24.6g
1 cup chopped kale	Fat: 2.3g
½ cup diced tomatoes	Carbohydrates: 65.2g
1 diced carrot and 1 diced celery stalk	Fiber: 20.7g
Seasonings: garlic, onion, thyme, salt, and pepper to taste	This warming soup offers a nutrient-dense option for your first meal, loaded with fiber, protein, and essential vitamins, making it perfect for a colder day or when you crave something comforting yet healthy.

Instructions:

1. In a large pot, sauté garlic and onion until softened.

2. Add diced carrots and celery, cooking until slightly tender.

3. Stir in the cooked lentils, chopped kale, and diced tomatoes, then pour in the vegetable broth.

4. Bring to a simmer and cook until the vegetables are tender and the flavors meld together.

5. Season with thyme, salt, and pepper.

Dinner 1: Grilled Chicken and Quinoa Salad

Ingredients: **Nutritional Value & Calories:**

4 oz grilled chicken breast   Calories: Approximately 618

1 cup cooked quinoa   Protein: 48.6g

2 cups mixed greens (like spinach)   Fat: 25.6g

½ cup cherry tomatoes, halved   Carbohydrates: 48.9g

¼ cucumber, sliced   Fiber: 7.7g

2 tablespoons feta cheese, crumbled   This protein-packed salad is not only
                                          filling but also combines a variety of
Dressing: Olive oil, lemon juice,   textures and flavors, along with a
minced garlic, salt, and pepper   healthy dose of calcium and fiber.

Instructions:

1. In a large bowl, mix the cooked quinoa with mixed greens, cherry tomatoes, and cucumber.

2. Slice the grilled chicken and add it to the salad.

3. Sprinkle with crumbled feta cheese.

4. Combine the dressing ingredients, adjust to taste, and drizzle over the salad.

Dinner 2: Baked Salmon with Roasted Vegetables

Ingredients:

Nutritional Value & Calories:

4 oz salmon fillet

1 cup broccoli florets

½ cup carrots, sliced

½ cup Brussels sprouts, halved

Olive oil, salt, and pepper for seasoning

A squeeze of lemon juice for flavor

Calories: Approximately 441

Protein: 30.2g

Fat: 28.9g

Carbohydrates: 18.3g

Fiber: 6.2g

This meal offers a hearty dose of omega-3 fatty acids, essential for heart and brain health, alongside a variety of vegetables for fiber and micronutrients.

Instructions:

1. Preheat the oven to 400°F (200°C).

2. Toss the broccoli, carrots, and Brussels sprouts in olive oil, salt, and pepper, and spread them on a baking sheet.

3. Place the salmon fillet among the vegetables.

4. Bake for 15-20 minutes, or until the salmon is cooked through and the vegetables are tender.

5. Finish with a squeeze of lemon juice over the salmon.

Dinner 3: Spinach and Ricotta Stuffed Portobello Mushrooms

Ingredients:

2 large Portobello mushroom caps, stems removed

1 cup ricotta cheese

1 cup spinach, chopped

¼ cup grated Parmesan cheese

1 garlic clove, minced

Salt, pepper, and Italian seasoning to taste

A drizzle of olive oil

Nutritional Value & Calories:

Calories: Approximately 727

Protein: 43.1g

Fat: 53.5g

Carbohydrates: 19.5g

Fiber: 2.8g

This dish combines the health benefits of spinach with the richness of ricotta and Parmesan, creating a satisfying and nutrient-rich dinner that's perfect for ending the eating window on a high note.

Instructions:

1. Preheat the oven to 375°F (190°C).

2. In a bowl, mix ricotta, spinach, Parmesan, garlic, salt, pepper, and Italian seasoning.

3. Place the mushroom caps on a baking sheet, gill-side up, and drizzle with olive oil.

4. Spoon the ricotta-spinach mixture into the mushrooms.

5. Bake for 20-25 minutes, or until the mushrooms are tender and the filling is heated through.

Bonus: Delicious Chia Seed Pudding Variations

Basic Chia Seed Pudding Recipe

Ingredients:

Nutritional Value & Calories:

1/4 cup chia seeds

Calories: Approximately 334

1 cup milk (any kind of milk will work, such as almond, coconut, soy, or cow's milk)

Protein: 9g

Fat: 17.5g

1-2 tablespoons maple syrup or honey, to taste

Carbohydrates: 34.5g

Fiber: 20g

1 teaspoon vanilla extract

This dish is ideal for those seeking a balanced, healthful option that supports sustained energy and provides significant health benefits.

Instructions:

1.   Mix Ingredients: In a bowl or mason jar, combine the chia seeds, milk, maple syrup (or honey), and vanilla extract. Stir well to mix everything thoroughly. Ensure the chia seeds are fully immersed in the liquid to avoid clumps.

2.   Refrigerate: Cover the bowl or close the jar, and place it in the refrigerator. Let it sit for at least 2 hours, though preferably overnight. This resting period allows the chia seeds to absorb the liquid and gel up, creating a pudding-like consistency.

3.   Stir and Serve: Once the chia seed pudding has thickened to your liking, give it a good stir to break up any clumps. If the pudding is too thick, you can add a bit more milk to adjust the consistency.

4.   Add Toppings: Serve the pudding with your choice of toppings. Popular options include fresh fruits (like berries, banana slices, or mango), nuts, coconut flakes, a dollop of yogurt, or a sprinkle of cinnamon.

Variation 1. Chocolate Chia Seed Pudding

Add 2 tablespoons of cocoa powder to the mixture before refrigerating. For a richer chocolate flavor and extra sweetness, mix in some chocolate chips or a drizzle of chocolate syrup before serving.

Variation 2. Berry Chia Seed Pudding

Blend 1/2 cup of your favorite berries (such as strawberries or blueberries) with the milk before mixing it with the chia seeds. This will give the pudding a fruity flavor and vibrant color.

Variation 3. Peanut Butter Banana Chia Seed Pudding

Mix 2 tablespoons of peanut butter into the pudding mixture before refrigerating. Serve with sliced bananas and a drizzle of honey for extra sweetness and flavor.

Variation 4. Kiwi-Banana Chia Seed Pudding

Use rice milk for the base, and don't use any sweeteners in case bananas and kiwi are very sweet. Make a purée from kiwi and banana using a blender, amounts depend on the size of the pudding you are preparing. Mix it all together with pudding before putting it into the refrigerator.

5 INTEGRATING INTERMITTENT FASTING INTO YOUR LIFESTYLE

More than merely changing one's diet, intermittent fasting is a way of life that has several potential health advantages. But in order for intermittent fasting to be really beneficial and long-lasting, it must be smoothly incorporated into every area of your life. This entails striking a balance between traveling, socializing, working out, and fasting.

Combining Intermittent Fasting with Exercise

Intermittent fasting and exercise complement each other well and can increase each other's advantages. When you exercise during your window of fasting can affect how you feel and function:

Fasted Exercise: Engaging in physical activity before your first meal can increase fat oxidation and improve metabolic adaptability. It's ideal for low to moderate-intensity workouts.

Fed Exercise: For more intense or longer-duration workouts, exercising after eating can help ensure you have enough energy, reducing the risk of fatigue and optimizing recovery.

For women over 50, balancing exercise types is key. A mix of cardiovascular exercises (for heart health), strength training (to combat muscle loss and support bone density), and flexibility or balance exercises (to enhance mobility and reduce injury risk) is recommended. We will discuss exercises during the intermittent fasting process further in Chapter 6.

Social Events and Eating Out

Social gatherings often revolve around meals, which can pose a challenge to maintaining your intermittent fasting schedule. Planning ahead is essential:

Adjust Your Fasting Window: If possible, adjust your fasting window on days you have social plans to accommodate meals out. You don't have to use the same method every week. Combining different methods may be difficult at the beginning, but with time you notice that your planning comes automatically and you don't need to overthink it.

Make Informed Food Choices: When eating out, opt for meals that align with your nutritional needs—high in protein, fiber, and healthy fats. Ask the waiter if there is a possibility to adjust the ordered meal according to your diet. If you eat in the company of people who don't know about your fasting, consider telling them about it. It may take away the pressure you can feel regarding your meal choice.

Enjoy Mindfully: Focus on the social experience rather than the food. Enjoying the company of friends and family can make adhering to your intermittent fasting plan more manageable. As scientists were studying the health of centenarians, they concluded, that eating while enjoying the company can saturate faster without overeating and give a boost for metabolism. It is said to be one of the reasons people live longer in close communities.

Fasting During Travel

Traveling can disrupt regular routines, making adherence to intermittent fasting more challenging. Consider your body condition when planning to integrate intermittent fasting with travel: sometimes it is not possible to combine them. For example, if you make a long-hour flight with catering on board, it would be unnecessary to refuse the meal. Catering on board is mostly very carefully planned and missing a meal could make you very hungry or nauseous.

To maintain your fasting schedule while on the move:

Plan Ahead: If you're flying, consider scheduling your travel during your fasting window, or if impossible, skip the day. For road trips, pack healthy snacks that fit within your eating window. Snacks like cheese, baby carrots, cucumber, fruits, or dried fruits and nuts are wonderful alternatives to unhealthy chips.

Stay Hydrated: Keep a water bottle handy, especially important during travel when it's easy to become dehydrated. The need for fluids is mostly higher during traveling, but it can also result in swollen feet and hands. For better blood circulation and other benefits like preventing thrombosis, use compression stockings.

Be Flexible: Allow yourself some flexibility with your fasting schedule to accommodate time zone changes and unique travel experiences. Remind yourself, that traveling is a stressful event for the whole body, so putting it more under pressure for not having followed the routine is unnecessary. There will be another day and another perfect moment to proceed with intermittent fasting.

Fasting and Work Conditions

From all recommendations on this topic, this would be the most difficult to make, as the work conditions can be different for different people even in the same place of work. There are some things to be considered:

Is my work plan constant or flexible?

Are my working days and hours the same in the week?

Do I have days when I am working from home or need to travel?

Do I have night shifts or different working shifts like mornings and evenings?

Do I have the possibility to prepare and consume food at work?

Do I have the possibility to take a break in times I need it?

Will I be under pressure if my colleagues will know about my intermittent fasting?

It can be very tricky and stressful to integrate intermittent fasting into your working routine. I was working in the hospital and my biggest issue was the night shift when I was supposed to work for 8 hours without food. As time went on, I adjusted my methods to working hours and immediately felt better and energized. From a medical point of view, it is not healthy to consume food in the hours when melatonin is the highest, so between 10 PM and 4 PM with its peak levels around 2 PM. As I started to break my fast around 5 AM I was able to finish my night shift with the needed amount of energy and had a restful sleep as my shift ended and I was home around 7 AM. I sincerely wish that you would also find the best approach, combining intermittent fasting with your working conditions.

6 EXERCISE RECOMMENDATIONS DURING INTERMITTENT FASTING

This chapter is dedicated to recommendations for exercises and physical activities during intermittent fasting. Note that those are general recommendations and for a more individual approach it is better to consult with a specialist, especially if you are new to sports and exercises. In case you have established your routine during your life, you can continue doing it while fasting. Adjust it according to your physical conditions and eating windows.

Understanding the Basics

The Importance of Exercise

Physical activity has an increasingly important role in preserving health and wellbeing as we age. Frequent exercise has several advantages, such as increased balance, flexibility, and strength. Exercise also lowers the risk of osteoporosis by promoting healthy bone density, which typically declines with age. Another important issue that regular physical activity can help with is cardiovascular health, which can improve circulation, lower blood pressure, and help avoid heart disease.

Exercise accelerates metabolism, which slows decreases as we age and aids in better control of body weight and composition. It also has a significant impact on mental health, helping to promote better mood, lessen anxiety and depressive symptoms, and improve cognitive performance. Engaging in regular physical activity helps older persons maintain their independence and enhances their quality of life by energizing everyday routines and reducing their dependence on others.

How Intermittent Fasting Affects Exercise Performance

It has been demonstrated that intermittent fasting affects exercise performance in a number of ways. When done properly, it can improve fat utilization and energy efficiency, which is advantageous for both resistance and aerobic training. Fasting intervals have the potential to enhance muscle tissue metabolic adaptations, increasing their capacity to use fat as an energy source. This is especially advantageous for extended or endurance-based exercise.

The timing of exercise, however, can have a big impact on recovery and performance during the fasting and feeding windows. Exercise during a fast period may accelerate fat loss and enhance metabolic health, but if done carelessly, it can also result in lower energy levels. It's critical to make sure that exercise is scheduled appropriately to help muscle regeneration and recovery by consuming nutrients throughout the feeding windows. After working exercise, eating a high-protein, high-carb meal as soon as possible can assist assure total recovery, repair muscle damage, and restore energy storage.

Types of Exercises Suitable for Women Over 50

Exercise for women over 50 should address specific physiological changes such as decreased bone density, reduced muscle mass, and the need for enhanced joint protection. Here, we explore a variety of exercise types that are particularly beneficial for women in this age group, focusing on cardiovascular health, strength maintenance, flexibility, and balance.

Cardiovascular Exercises

Cardiovascular exercise is vital for heart health, weight management, and metabolic function. Activities such as walking, swimming, and cycling are excellent options. These low-impact exercises are easier on the joints while effectively boosting heart rate and improving circulation.

Walking: A simple yet powerful exercise that can be easily incorporated into daily routines. It's accessible, requires no special equipment, and can be adjusted in intensity.

Swimming: Known for being gentle on the body, swimming provides a full-body workout that enhances cardiovascular health without putting stress on joints.

Cycling: Either stationary or on a bike, cycling is another low-impact cardiovascular workout that helps build leg strength and endurance while protecting the joints.

HIIT and REHIIT: High-Intensity Interval Training (HIIT) and Reduced Exertion High-Intensity Interval Training (REHIIT) are both fitness methodologies designed to achieve significant health and fitness benefits in short periods of training.

Strength Training

Strength training is crucial to counteract the natural loss of muscle mass and bone density that occurs with aging. Incorporating resistance training into an exercise routine can help maintain muscle strength, support metabolic health, and improve bone density.

Resistance Bands: These offer a versatile and joint-friendly way to perform strength training. They provide resistance without the impact of heavy weights, making them ideal for home workouts.

Weight Training: Using light to moderate weights can help build and maintain muscle mass. Exercises can include free weights, machines, or body weight. Best made under the surveillance of the fitness trainer.

Pilates: It is a low-impact exercise system that focuses on strengthening muscles while improving postural alignment and flexibility. Developed by Joseph Pilates in the early 20th century, it combines controlled movements and breathing to enhance body awareness, core strength, and overall stability. Pilates exercises are performed either on a mat or using specialized equipment, such as a reformer, which offers resistance for muscle toning and strength. The practice emphasizes precision and flow rather than intensity and high impact, making it suitable for people of all ages and fitness levels. Pilates is particularly beneficial for improving core strength, enhancing flexibility, and aiding in injury prevention and rehabilitation.

Flexibility and Balance Exercises

Maintaining flexibility and balance is essential for preventing falls. Exercises that enhance these attributes can help maintain independence and mobility.

Yoga: It is an ancient physical, mental, and spiritual practice that originated in India over 5,000 years ago. It encompasses a broad range of techniques, including physical postures (asanas), breathing exercises (pranayama), meditation, and ethical precepts. Yoga is designed to improve physical health, promote emotional wellbeing, enhance mental clarity, and foster spiritual growth. Its practice can range from gentle and restorative to highly vigorous and physically demanding, making it accessible and beneficial for individuals of all ages and fitness levels. The diversity of yoga styles and practices allows it to be tailored to personal preferences and needs, contributing to its widespread popularity as a holistic approach to health and wellness.

Tai Chi: A traditional Chinese martial art known for its slow, fluid movements and deep breathing techniques. Often described as "meditation in motion," Tai Chi promotes physical balance, flexibility, and cardiovascular fitness, while also reducing stress and improving mental focus. The gentle and deliberate movements of Tai Chi are designed to foster a calm mind and a healthy body by enhancing the flow of "Qi" (vital energy) throughout the body.

Practiced worldwide by people of all ages, Tai Chi is especially popular among older adults due to its low-impact nature and numerous health benefits, including improved balance, enhanced muscular strength, and greater overall psychological wellbeing.

Qigong: Traditional Chinese mind-body practice that combines movement, meditation, and controlled breathing to enhance physical and mental wellbeing. The word "qigong" translates to "life energy cultivation" and is designed to help balance and harness the body's vital energy, or "qi." Qigong exercises involve rhythmic movements, focused breathing, and mindful meditation, often practiced to improve health, increase vitality, and promote the circulation of qi throughout the body. The practice of qigong is rooted in traditional Chinese medicine, martial arts, and philosophy, offering a holistic approach to health maintenance and healing. It is characterized by gentle, flowing movements that are typically easy to learn and can be adapted to fit any age or fitness level, making it particularly popular among those seeking a gentle form of exercise that emphasizes inner peace and physical balance.

Aqua Aerobics: Aqua aerobics, or water aerobics, is an excellent low-impact exercise, providing a host of health benefits in a buoyant, water-based environment. The water's natural resistance ensures that muscles work harder without stressing the joints, making it ideal for those with arthritis or osteoporosis. This form of exercise enhances cardiovascular health, boosts muscle strength, improves flexibility and balance, and aids in weight management—all critical for aging bodies. Additionally, exercising in water prevents overheating and offers a calming effect, reducing stress and improving mental health. Aqua aerobics is adaptable to all fitness levels, making it a versatile and accessible option for maintaining health and enhancing the quality of life as women age.

Benefits of Restorative Yoga

We spoke shortly about yoga and its diversity, but there is one yoga style that is particularly beneficial for all women regardless of age. It is a restorative yoga, known under the name of yin yoga.

Yin yoga is a slow-paced style of yoga that involves holding passive poses for longer periods, typically between three to five minutes or even longer. This form of yoga aims to apply moderate stress to the connective tissues—the tendons, fascia, and ligaments—to increase circulation in the joints and improving flexibility. By relaxing the muscles and holding the poses for extended durations, Yin yoga facilitates deeper access to the body's deeper connective tissues.

This gentle form of yoga uses props like bolsters, blankets, and blocks to support the body in various poses, which facilitates deeper relaxation and healing. The key benefits of this type of exercise are enhanced flexibility and mobility, improved stress and balance, stress reduction and mental clarity, better sleep quality, hormonal balance, pain and chronic condition management and strengthening of pelvic floor muscles.

Pelvic Floor Exercises

An essential component of the body's core are the pelvic floor muscles. Any physical activity benefits from improved core stability and alignment, which is what strengthening them brings. Better posture and balance come from having a strong core, which also leads to more effective movement patterns during exercise that increase stamina and decrease tiredness. When breathing, the pelvic floor muscles cooperate with the diaphragm. Breathing efficiency can be increased and the diaphragm supported by a robust pelvic floor. Improved breathing results in improved oxygen exchange, which is essential for physical activity-related endurance and stamina.

Lower back and pelvic injuries are less likely when there is a strong pelvic floor because it stabilizes the pelvis during physical activity. Maintaining continuous training and performance is dependent upon injury prevention, which has a positive impact on vitality.

Having a strong pelvic floor also helps with sexual function, which indirectly improves general energy and endurance. Better blood flow and muscular control can increase vitality and general well-being, which can lead to increased endurance in a variety of spheres of life.

Regular pelvic floor exercises are a vital part of any comprehensive fitness program, but they are especially important for people who want to improve their endurance and physical performance.

Restorative Yoga Poses

Restorative yoga poses are typically held for longer periods, ranging from 5 to 20 minutes, to allow practitioners to sink into deep relaxation and achieve a meditative state. At the beginning, you may start with 2 minutes or even 30 seconds, and you should always listen to your body. If you feel pleasant stretch and relax with every breath. If the pain is unbearable, go out of the pose and try something other.

Here are some common forms or types of poses used in restorative yoga:

Supported Backbends

These poses open up the chest and heart area, which can be therapeutic for improving respiratory functions and alleviating mild depression or anxiety. Props like bolsters, blankets, and blocks are used to support the back, allowing the chest to open gently without strain. You can put your feet on the ground, or straighten them. A butterfly pole with feet soles touching each other is also a variation.

Example: Supported Bridge Pose

A bolster or several folded blankets are placed under the sacrum to gently elevate the hips, allowing the spine to arch naturally over the base of support.

Supported Forward Bends

These poses promote a sense of calm and help to soothe the nervous system by encouraging inward focus and deep breathing. They are particularly beneficial for cooling down the body and quieting the mind.

Example: Supported Child's Pose

Cushions or a bolster are placed between the legs, and the torso rests downward, with the forehead supported by additional padding if necessary.

Supported Inversions

Inversions like legs up the wall are part of restorative yoga that help in reversing the blood flow and relieving tired legs and feet. They can also help in calming the nervous system.

Example: Legs-Up-The-Wall Pose

The legs are extended vertically up a wall while the back rests flat on the floor, often with a bolster supporting the hips to elevate them slightly.

Supine Poses

These poses are performed lying on the back and are excellent for deeply relaxing the body. They can include slight twists or simply lying flat with limbs supported.

Example: Corpse Pose

The body lies flat on the back, perhaps with a bolster under the knees, a rolled blanket under the neck, and eye pillows over the eyes to promote complete relaxation.

Gentle Twists

Gentle twists help in releasing tension from the spine and abdominal organs. In restorative yoga, these twists are performed very gently with plenty of support to avoid any strain.

Example: Thread the Needle Pose

Begin on all fours, ensuring your knees are under your hips and your wrists are under your shoulders. Inhale and reach your right arm up toward the ceiling, opening your chest while keeping your hips squared and stable. This is a gentle opening twist for the upper back.

As you exhale, slowly thread your right arm under your left arm, bringing your right shoulder and cheek gently down to the mat. Your left arm can remain extended forward or, for a deeper stretch, you can wrap it around your back toward your right thigh. Stay in this position for 5-10 breaths, focusing on relaxing into the pose and allowing the tension in your shoulders and upper back to release. The weight of your body should be evenly distributed to avoid strain. Repeat the same sequence on the left side.

Each of these restorative poses focuses on relaxation, recovery, and gentle stretching. The key is to create a comfortable environment where the body can rest deeply while the mind unwinds. This form of yoga is particularly beneficial for reducing stress and anxiety, aiding digestion, improving sleep, and overall wellbeing.

Trying Out Alternative Physical Activities

Some physical activities are more like hobbies than sports but still can be beneficial for metabolism and overall health. These alternatives are often more flexible, accessible, and varied, catering to individual preferences and needs. Here are some popular options:

Walking: One of the simplest forms of exercise, walking can be done almost anywhere and adjusted in pace and distance to suit fitness levels. It's excellent for cardiovascular health, weight management, and reducing the risk of chronic diseases.

Dancing: Dance is also a form of fitness, that brings a lot of joy and a feeling of emotional release. Dancing in fitness classes or simply dancing to music at home can be a fun and effective way to get a cardiovascular workout, improve balance, and increase flexibility.

Hiking: Hiking not only provides a cardiovascular workout but also offers mental health benefits associated with being in nature. It can be a more strenuous form of walking, often involving varied terrain that challenges the body in different ways.

Gardening: Surprisingly physical, gardening involves bending, lifting, digging, and stretching, providing a moderate-intensity workout that can improve endurance, strength, and flexibility.

Dog walking: Caring for the dogs as pets may bring a lot of fun and movement every day. The dogs are perfect buddies for walking and physical activities outside. However, it should not be the only reason for taking a dog, as they need a lot of care and affliction.

Playing: More and more scientific researchers are interested in the benefits of playing. Physical play, including activities like team sports, games, and recreational exercises, offers numerous benefits, contributing significantly to physical health, mental wellbeing, and social interactions. Physical play stimulates the release of endorphins, the body's natural mood elevators. This can reduce feelings of depression and anxiety. Additionally, engaging in playful activities can improve cognitive functions by keeping the brain active and engaged, potentially delaying the onset of cognitive decline and promoting overall brain health.

Cleaning: No matter how funny or frustrating it may feel, cleaning is a wonderful calorie burner. Engaging in household chores can turn into a surprising fitness session, especially for those looking for easy ways to fit more physical activity into their day. Cleaning activities require body movement over a range of motions, engaging multiple muscle groups. Depending on the intensity and your body weight, you can burn approximately 150 to 300 calories per hour.

Connection Between Lymph Fluid and Weight

The Invisible Fluid

Lymph fluid and the lymphatic system play crucial roles in maintaining overall health, including influencing weight management. The lymphatic system, a critical part of the body's immune and circulatory systems, is responsible for transporting lymph, a fluid containing white blood cells that help fight infection.

The lymphatic system helps to remove excess fluids from body tissues. If the lymphatic system is sluggish or inefficient, it can lead to fluid retention, contributing to swelling and a temporary increase in body weight. This is often noticeable in conditions like lymphedema, where lymphatic drainage is impaired, causing significant swelling in body parts like limbs. Cellulitis on the thighs is one of the most famous symptoms of stagnation of lymphatic flow and can be significantly improved with lymphatic drainage techniques in the hip and groin area.

The lymphatic system assists in transporting waste and toxins away from the tissues and into the circulatory system to be expelled from the body. Poor lymphatic circulation can hinder this process, potentially contributing to the buildup of fat deposits and toxins, which can affect metabolism and weight management. Many people experience immediate weight improvement already after a few sessions of lymphatic massage or exercises found on the internet.

Lymphatic Drainage

Lymphatic drainage is a therapeutic massage technique designed to stimulate the flow of lymph fluid. It can also be part of a wellness routine to support a healthy immune system and manage inflammation.

Lymphatic drainage involves gentle, rhythmic massage movements that follow the direction of the body's lymphatic flow. The aim is to enhance the natural drainage of lymph, which carries waste products away from the tissues and back toward the heart. This type of massage is particularly beneficial for reducing swelling, detoxifying the body, improving circulation, and potentially helping with weight loss by enhancing metabolic rate as the body more efficiently removes waste and balances fluid levels.

Benefits of Fascia Treatment

Fascia is a band or sheet of connective tissue, primarily made up of collagen, that lies beneath the skin. It attaches, stabilizes, encloses, and separates interior organs and muscles. The use of fascia (or massage) balls in fascia treatment has grown in popularity due to its many physical advantages, especially in terms of increasing mobility, decreasing pain, and boosting general body function.

Increased blood flow to various body parts is one of the benefits of fascia therapy. Improved circulation can help remove metabolic waste more quickly by supplying tissues with more oxygen and nutrients. This increased blood flow has the potential to hasten recovery and lessen post-workout discomfort.

Regular fascia therapy helps relax and release tight fascia, increasing the body's general range of motion and flexibility. For people who are stiff or participate in activities requiring a lot of range of motion, this is quite helpful.

These treatments can reduce chronic pain issues associated with muscle imbalances and restricted fascia movement by dissolving scar tissue and relaxing tight fascia. It works very well for some types of back pain. Fascia therapy can enhance muscular balance and biomechanical efficiency in athletes. Enhancement of performance and decreased risk of injury can be achieved by the release of tension and limitations in the fascia.

Fascia therapy can help with recovery from intense physical activity by assisting in the dispersal of the acid products of exercise that accumulate in the muscles, which frequently causes discomfort and microscopic tears in the muscle fibers.

Benefits of Fascia Balls

Fascia balls are tools designed to target specific areas of the body for fascia release. They can target smaller or more specific areas that are difficult to reach with larger rollers or other tools. This makes them particularly effective for deep tissue manipulation and for accessing trigger points. Due to their size and ease of use, fascia balls are highly portable and can be used anywhere. Whether at home, in the office, or while traveling, users can perform essential fascia releases without the need for professional help. Having a fascia ball or even a tennis ball on a long flight or even during a conference can significantly reduce pain in the back, shoulders, and neck.

By adjusting the amount of body weight used, you can customize the pressure to suit the comfort level and specific needs. This adaptability makes fascia balls suitable for a wide range of users, from athletes to those with chronic pain. Fascia balls are a cost-effective solution for ongoing self-maintenance, reducing the need for frequent professional massage or physical therapy sessions. The only thing you need is to purchase a variety of fascia balls, rollers, or even just tennis balls and research some exercises and positioning

70

recommendations on the internet.

Timing Your Workouts with Fasting

Integrating exercise into an intermittent fasting schedule poses unique challenges and opportunities. Understanding how to properly time workouts during fasting periods can maximize both fat loss and muscle preservation, while also ensuring that energy levels are maintained. This subchapter explores strategies for synchronizing exercise with fasting, enhancing performance, and optimizing recovery.

Understanding Energy Dynamics

The body's energy dynamics shift significantly during fasting. Initially, glycogen stores in the liver and muscles are used as the primary energy source. As fasting continues, these stores deplete, and the body increases fat oxidation, using fat as its primary fuel source. Timing exercises during these phases can leverage these energy shifts for improved fitness results.

Exercising During Glycogen Depletion: Engaging in aerobic activities such as walking or light cycling during the later stages of a fasting period can enhance fat burning, as the body transitions to using fat for fuel.

Strength Training and Glycogen Availability: For resistance training, which typically relies on glycogen, it may be more effective to schedule workouts soon after a meal when glycogen stores are replenished.

Workout Timing Strategies

Optimal timing for exercise during intermittent fasting varies depending on the fasting schedule and the type of exercise:

Morning Workouts: For those who skip breakfast, engaging in light to moderate exercise in the morning can be effective. This timing takes advantage of the hormonal milieu—typically higher cortisol and growth hormone levels—that supports fat metabolism.

Postprandial Workouts: Exercising after the first meal of the day can be ideal, especially for more intense or longer-duration workouts. This timing ensures that energy levels are supported by food intake, which is critical for maintaining intensity and preventing muscle loss.

Adjusting Exercise Intensity

During fasting, particularly if it is a longer duration, it may be necessary to adjust exercise intensity. It is especially needed if you are new to a fitness routine.

Reduced Intensity: When fully fasted, consider reducing the intensity of workouts to accommodate decreased energy availability and to prevent undue fatigue.

Increased Intensity Post-Meal: After eating, the body's increased glucose availability makes it an ideal time to engage in higher-intensity or resistance-based workouts.

Recovery Considerations

Light activities such as stretching, yoga, or walking on rest days can enhance circulation and aid in recovery without overly taxing the body's energy reserves.

It is also important to adjust recovery strategies to fit within the fasting framework. Consume a meal rich in protein and carbohydrates soon after strength training to aid in muscle recovery and growth. This meal should ideally fall within the eating window to maximize recovery. Also wisely chosen protein shakes can serve as a meal substitute, but not for every day and it should be not more than once a day.

Listening to Your Body

As stated earlier, adjusting both the timing and type of exercise based on personal energy levels and health status is vital. It might sound already boring, but beginners should consider consulting with health professionals to tailor the exercise and fasting regimen, so they can ensure that it aligns with individual health needs and fitness goals..

Safety Tips and Injury Prevention

Exercising is one thing, but exercising safely is another: it is crucial to avoid injuries and ensure a long-term, sustainable fitness routine. As the body changes over time, it becomes more susceptible to injuries due to decreased bone density, reduced muscle mass, and less elastic tendons and ligaments. It mam and may not happen to you, as everybody´s constitution is individual.

Warm-Up and Cool-Down Routines

Incorporating comprehensive warm-up and cool-down routines is essential, so your general exercise routine won´t bring your body and muscles into shock.

Begin every exercise session with at least 5-10 minutes of light aerobic activity to increase blood flow to the muscles and reduce the risk of injury. Follow this with dynamic stretches to improve the range of motion and prepare the body for the workout. Listen to your body and even if you follow a special everyday routine, your body needs may change and some exercises might not be suitable on a particular day.

End each session with a cool-down period that gradually reduces the heart rate to its resting state. Include static stretches to improve flexibility and decrease muscle stiffness, consider implementing a few yin yoga exercises, especially those for open and mobile hips.

Don't forget about rest and recovery: allow adequate recovery time between workouts, especially after more intense sessions. Adequate sleep and rest days are important for muscle repair and overall recovery. It is not necessary to do fitness every day of the week. Muscles need time to recover and regenerate, so

2-3 times a week is a good starting point. Your routine doesn't have to be long either: starting from 20 minutes it can be already very efficient.

Exercise Modification and Equipment

As mentioned earlier, every day is a different day and your body changes constantly. Modifying and changing exercises to reduce strain on joints and muscles could be a good idea, or even changing your routine according to muscle group or body area that needs special attention. For example, replace high-impact exercises like running with low-impact activities such as walking or swimming, or in case of dizziness try out slow and dynamic exercises and exercises for balance.

Appropriate Equipment is another important thing. Use proper workout gear, especially footwear that provides adequate support and cushioning. Also, consider using assistive devices as needed, such as wrist wraps or knee braces. It could be overwhelming to find all the needed information about equipment, but there are tons of information on the Internet and you always can ask for assistance in sports shops.

Technique and Posture

If you are new to a fitness routine, there is another thing that I would like to tell you about and you might ever know it very well. It is not always easy to follow instructors online or in the courses, because sometimes we don't feel and see how our body moves and adjusts to the exercise. However, maintaining correct form and posture during exercises is vital, as a wrongly positioned body during exercise may damage your muscles or spine.

It's beneficial to work with a fitness professional who can instruct on the correct form and technique for various exercises, particularly when using weights or performing complex movements. If possible, film yourself while doing some difficult or new exercises, to watch and adjust it afterward, or to compare with those made by the instructor. Mirror is another good option.

7 BEING AWARE OF YOUR BODY, MIND AND SOUL

This chapter of the book is one of my favorite ones. As a natural seeker for perfect wellbeing, I came to understand that our body, mind, and soul have to be in balance. Finding this balance is a lifetime of work, but it is often interesting and pays itself off in a positive matter.

The Power of Meditation

It is believed that meditation is something to be learned and practiced regularly. When one thinks about meditation, pictures like sitting in the lotus pose come into mind, or laying down with closed eyes. In reality, meditation surrounds us every day and in every possible situation: during the walk, sleep, praying, contemplating in the car, doing makeup, or preparing dinner. This state is an in-born state and we don't need to learn something we came with into this world. Nevertheless, the modern world makes timing for meditation difficult to find, and we are trying to grasp with logical minds what meditation is and how to reach different steps of it. At the same time now is the most needed time on earth, for people to remember how to meditate and contemplate.

Benefits of Meditation

Meditation offers profound benefits for both mental and physical health. Psychologically, it helps reduce stress, anxiety, and depression by promoting a state of relaxation and presence. Regular practice leads to improved focus, better memory, and greater emotional resilience. Physically, meditation can lower blood pressure, reduce chronic pain, and enhance sleep quality.

Types of Meditation

There are countless types of meditation as a relaxation technique to name. For example, breathing techniques, music, taking a bath, and so on. I would like to recommend some of the methods that I use and see the benefits of it in my clients.

Guided Meditations: Perfect for beginners and not only. Especially good if there is a subject or theme to meditate on. YouTube is full of videos on different subjects, in every length possible.

Guided Sleep Hypnosis: An amazing tool for overcoming mind-made obstacles in achieving goals. For example, Michael Sealey gives wonderful hypnosis for enchanting weight loss, overcoming binge eating, etc.

Mindfulness Meditations: Mindfulness involves paying full attention to the present moment without judgment. This can be practiced throughout the day, whether you're eating, walking, or simply breathing. By observing sensations, thoughts, and emotions as they arise, mindfulness fosters a greater understanding of one's mental and emotional patterns, leading to increased patience and compassion. The best mindfulness meditation is just observing your breath pattern, without any goals or judgment.

Breathing Meditations: Similar to mindfulness meditation, but proposing tens of different breathing techniques from around the world, may change your mood and condition literally in a few minutes. You can address many issues with breathing, for example, panic attacks or overheating. The Internet gives a lot of information on that subject.

Being in Nature: Gardening, walking or just watching the trees and the birds are also a form of meditation. Closing your eyes and picturing that the wind speaks to you, or speaking with the earth you are cultivating: the is a lot of magic that cannot be described, but can only be felt.

Using the Apps: In times of IT growth and expansion, there are probably different applications for different issues. One of my favorite applications for meditation is Triple Flame from Gene Keys founder Richard Rudd. You can adjust the timer on how many times in the day you want to meditate and it will remind you. App hat amazing materials and audios, and very relaxing music.

Listening to Different Frequency Music

As we know from physics, everything has its frequency and vibration. Different cells of our body, emotions, or every ailment have their frequency. Listening to music with those specific frequencies can bring forth changes in your whole system. For example, for quick recharge, I love listening to Schumann's Resonance. At the beginning I needed to listen to that recording for at least an hour to feel energized, but as time went by I took something between 7-11 minutes.

Mantras and Chanting: coming from Indian Vedic tradition, this technique is similar to vocal praying in Western culture. Reciting the same words over and over again brings a sense of calmness, peace, and tranquility. Alternatively, you may use any affirmations and intentions, and repeat them as long as you feel it is needed.

Integrating Meditation into Daily Life

Incorporating meditation into daily life can seem challenging, but even a few minutes a day can make a significant difference. It is more beneficial to meditate for a few minutes every day than to meditate for a long period once or twice a week. Start with just five minutes in the morning or evening and gradually increase the duration, maybe even while you are still in bed or making your coffee.

It is nice to establish a specific place in your home for meditation, but it is not necessary. I enjoy meditating in my bed or on my couch and I don't have a special place for that. Also, many find meditating with a group more effective. This could be through a local meditation center or an online community.

Meditation is a deeply personal experience, and its practice can be adapted to fit one's lifestyle and preferences. To meditate or to not meditate - it is your own choice. But I assure you, you will enjoy enhanced mental clarity, emotional stability, and overall wellbeing, all of which are essential for a balanced and healthy life.

Conscious Eating and Emotions

These are other interesting subjects worth speaking about. There is a lot of information in this book about when to eat and what to eat, but now it´s time to speak about how to eat.

Being Conscious while Eating

In our busy world stress levels may be so high that we want to escape them by watching TV, scrolling social media posts, telephoning with someone, etc. It all might be okay if happens once or twice, but I don't recommend practicing it every time you take a meal in. We tend to eat more or stay hungry if we are not aware of our eating, as our consciousness dwells elsewhere and we are not present. The practitioners of intuitive eating state, that a person should stop eating if he feels that his stomach is about 80 percent full. This feeling is impossible to perceive if we constantly put our awareness into some distraction.

Imagine cooking yourself a nice and tasty dinner. You´ve spent some time in the kitchen, preparing food for the most important person in your life: yourself. Yes, indeed, you and your body are the most important on this journey. Every organ and every cell deserves to be treated with love, importance, attention, and care. So, make eating your personal meditation,

76

make it a love and gratitude ritual, and enjoy every bite you take!

Working with Emotions

The journey of intermittent fasting will not always be sweet like honey. There will be days full of obstacles, emotional roller coasters, and feelings you may never experienced before in your life.

There is one technique I once read about, the source of which I cannot remember anymore. I have adjusted it for myself and would like to share it with you.

Imagine a moment, when you experience emotion that makes you feel strange and uncomfortable. For example, you have a fear that your partner will laugh at your plan to start with intermittent fasting. There is nothing you can change about your partner, but there is something you can do in yourself: transform and let go of your fear and detach from this feeling so it won´t bother you anymore.

This is what I do:

ALLOW this feeling to grow bigger and bigger, let it expand until it consumes you entirely.

ACCEPT this feeling. By doing so, you are "framing" it and stopping its expansion.

EMBRACE this feeling. Imagine as if this feeling is just a piece of paper that you are crumpling and making smaller so it could fit into your embrace.

RELEASE this feeling. Do not hold onto it anymore, just observe it from a distance feeling neutral.

LET GO of this feeling. You may observe it to go away in every direction you want: into the ground, to the sky, far away behind the horizon. Now breathe out and check if this feeling still bothers you.

You may repeat this exercise several times. Some emotions are rooted very deep inside us and one exercise might not bring the expected results. Our fears are lying deep like the center of the onion: we have to peel off layer by layer until we eventually get there.

8 TESTIMONIALS

Testimonial 1: Jane's Journey to Renewed Energy

"At 52, I felt as though my energy levels were declining every day, and the weight just kept creeping up, no matter what I tried. That's when I stumbled upon intermittent fasting. Initially skeptical, I started with a simple 14:10 method, gradually moving to 16:8 as my body adapted. The first few weeks were challenging, especially the morning hunger pangs, but I persisted. Remarkably, not only did I start losing weight, but my energy throughout the day skyrocketed. It's been six months, and I've lost 20 pounds. More importantly, I feel like I've regained my zest for life. Intermittent fasting has taught me the importance of listening to my body and nourishing it right. It's not just a diet; it's a lifestyle that I intend to maintain."

Testimonial 2: Maria's Metabolic Makeover

"After menopause, I noticed my metabolism wasn't what it used to be. I was gaining weight, especially around the midsection, and no amount of exercise seemed to help. When a friend introduced me to intermittent fasting, I was intrigued but cautious. At 57, I wasn't sure if it was the right move. However, after consulting with my doctor, I decided to give the 16:8 method a try. The results were astonishing. Not only did I start shedding the stubborn weight, but my blood sugar levels, which had been inching towards the pre-diabetic range, normalized. Intermittent fasting has been a game-changer for me. It's not always easy, especially during social events, but the benefits far outweigh the inconvenience. I feel healthier and more in control of my body than I have in years."

Testimonial 3: Susan's Strength and Serenity

"I've always been active, but as I approached my 50s, I noticed a decrease in my strength and an increase in joint pains. I was intrigued by potential benefits of intermittent fasting for inflammation and overall health. With a cautious start to the 5:2 method, where I ate normally for five days and reduced my calorie intake significantly for two days, I embarked on this new journey. The first month was a mix of trial and error, but with persistence, I began to notice changes. My joint pain diminished, and I felt stronger, both mentally and physically. It's been a year now, and I can confidently say that intermittent fasting has not only improved my physical health but has also brought a new level of calmness and resilience to my life. My advice to anyone considering intermittent fasting, especially women over 50, is to start slowly, be patient with yourself, and enjoy the journey to better health."

These testimonials highlight the diverse benefits and experiences of women over 50 who have embraced intermittent fasting. Whether it's seeking energy, metabolic health, or strength and wellbeing, intermittent fasting offers a flexible approach to health that can be adapted to meet individual needs and goals.

9 LOOKING FORWARD

As the practice of intermittent fasting continues to gain popularity and recognition for its myriad health benefits, individuals embarking on this journey will find it increasingly vital to stay informed and motivated. This chapter delves into the future of intermittent fasting research, provides guidance on continuing your intermittent fasting journey, and offers advice on staying informed and motivated.

The Future of Intermittent Fasting Research

Intermittent fasting has emerged as a significant area of nutritional research, with studies increasingly focusing on its long-term effects and potential health benefits beyond weight loss. Future research aims to unravel how fasting intervals affect metabolic pathways, brain health, aging processes, and chronic disease prevention. There is also a growing interest in personalized fasting methods, adapting fasting schedules to individual genetic profiles, lifestyles, and health conditions. As more comprehensive data becomes available, we can expect refined guidelines that cater to diverse populations, enhancing the efficacy and safety of intermittent fasting.

Continuing Your Journey with Intermittent Fasting

Continuing with intermittent fasting over the long term requires a blend of adaptability and consistency. As life circumstances and body responses change, so too should your fasting regimen. It's essential to regularly assess how your body responds to your current fasting plan and make adjustments as needed. This could mean altering fasting durations or the type of fasting to better suit your health needs and goals. Please check the worksheets at the end of the book for additional support. It is also totally fine to set new goals along the way: our consciousness and body awareness change every day and tomorrow our goals might not be as right as they were feeling today.

I also want to note again, that regular check-ins with healthcare providers can help tailor your fasting plan based on health screening results and nutritional needs. Having a professional on your side can give extra support and trust in the whole process and yourself.

Staying Informed and Motivated

Staying motivated and well-informed are key components of a successful intermittent fasting experience. To maintain enthusiasm and ensure safety, I recommend to consider the following strategies:

Educational Resources: Keep up-to-date with the latest intermittent fasting research and insights by reading books, reputable online resources, and scientific publications. Knowledge is not only empowering but also instrumental in refining and optimizing your fasting approach. I use the method of three sources: you collect the information from 3 sources and then decide, what information is useful and right for YOU.

Community Engagement: Join intermittent fasting forums, online groups, or local meetups where experiences, tips, and encouragement are shared. Being part of a community can provide a significant motivational boost and a sense of belonging. It might be easier to find the community online as in the local area, or you can consider starting your community and inviting others.

Incorporate Technology: Use apps and tracking tools to monitor your fasting windows, dietary intake, and health metrics. These tools can provide insightful feedback, help maintain discipline, and adjust your fasting plans effectively. Likely we have enough tools and apps for journeys like intermittent fasting or even for staying hydrated. It makes the whole process more fun and playful and serves as a reminder of the busy day.

The journey with intermittent fasting is both personal and dynamic. As research evolves and more is understood about the benefits and methods of intermittent fasting, you can adapt and refine your approach. By staying informed, engaged, and motivated, you can continue to reap the health benefits of intermittent fasting and ensure that it remains a sustainable and positive aspect of your lifestyle. I truly believe in you!

CONCLUSION

I want to take a moment here as we wrap up this extensive tutorial on intermittent fasting to honor the adventure you are about to start on or continue on. A better awareness of your body's demands and rhythms can be attained through intermittent fasting, which is more than just a dietary decision. The ideas and methods presented in this book are intended to help you reach your goals.

Recall that your intermittent fasting journey is unique to you. It's about figuring out a rhythm that suits your body, your lifestyle, and your health goals. There will be days when the fasting feels more difficult and the results don't seem to be happening right away, but as you get more aware of how your body reacts to various fasting periods and foods, keep an open mind and be curious. Accept the encouraging environment of other fasters, and don't be afraid to ask healthcare providers for advice on how to customize this experience to meet your unique health requirements.

I want you to remember the joy and hope that accompany starting or continuing a journey of transformation as you go forward. Honor each tiny accomplishment, each new understanding of your habits and health, and each progress. These are the experiences that deserve taking the trip.

Thank you for trusting this guide as a companion in your intermittent fasting journey. May this experience bring you not just the health outcomes you seek, but a greater joy and appreciation for the body that carries you through every day. Here's to your health, happiness, and a fulfilling fasting journey!

APPENDICES

Worksheet 1. Before Beginning

1. Do I have enough knowledge about intermittent fasting and am I ready to start?

2. What are my goals and intentions?

3. What feelings arise when I think about starting?

4. If those are positive feelings, which and why?

5. If those are negative feelings, which and why?

6. Do I want or need to tell my friends/family about my plan?

7. What reactions I can expect if I tell them about it?

8. Would those reactions influence me and my emotions/motivation?

9. If yes, why you think it would?

10. Do I have knowledge and skills how to manage stressful situations during fasting?

11. If yes, what are my best techniques I can use?

Worksheet 2. Preparation

1. Am I aware of my body health and fitness condition? Do I need to consult with healthcare provider before starting?

2. Are my living space/cupboards and fridge in the kitchen ready (if you feel decluttering necessary)?

3. Do I know which method to start with?

If no, consider reading additional information, consulting with healthcare provider or speaking with people who have experience with intermittent fasting.

4. Do I need or want to integrate physical activity into my intermittent fasting journey? If yes, what options I consider?

Worksheet 3. Lifestyle

1. Which method I find more suitable for my work/sleep schedule?

2. Do I have family commitments or eating traditions that I want to keep taking part of?

3. Do I take medications that are strongly connected with food intake?

4. Do I have health issues that hunger can trigger if fasting break too long? (For example, sugar levels, stomach acidity).

5. What are my food preparation and food intake possibilities at home and/or at work?

Worksheet 4. Self-Reflection before starting

1. How I think I will be able to manage hunger?

2. Do I believe in my goal?

3. Do I find my goal realistic?

4. How will I measure my achievements?

5. What message I want to give myself before I start?

Worksheet 5. Self-Reflection for every week

1. How was I managing hunger?

2. Did I had stressful days when I thought I won´t make it?

3. Did I had days when I had to break the fast?

4. What emotional conditions I experienced this week?

5. Is the method I chose working for me or I had to make adjustments?

6. What physical changes I experienced this week?

7. What resonance I experienced in my community about my fasting?

8. What do I wish to myself for the next week?

9. Please express gratitude for your achievements and progress.

Worksheet 6. Self-Reflection when achieving the goal

1. How do I feel after finishing this journey physically?

2. How do I feel emotionally?

3. How do I feel mentally?

4. What general experience I had with intermittent fasting?

5. Those are 3 challenges I had on my way.

6. Those are 3 positive things I had on my way.

7. Is my goal fully achieved?

8. Did I had to do adjustments for my goal?

9. If I would start this journey again, what would I say to myself?

10. Please express gratitude for your achievements and progress. Well done!

Worksheet 7. Working with emotions

The emotion and feeling I experience now is:

Why do I think this feeling came to surface? What triggered it?

Please follow those instructions. You can say it at loud if you wish.

I ALLOW this feeling to be. (Let it grow bigger and bigger, and expand until it consumes you entirely).

I ACCEPT this feeling. (By doing so, you are "framing" it and stopping its expansion).

I EMBRACE this feeling. (Imagine as if this feeling is just a piece of paper that you are crumpling and making smaller so it could fit into your embrace).

I RELEASE this feeling. (Do not hold onto it anymore, just observe it from a distance feeling neutral).

I LET GO of this feeling. (You may observe it to go away in every direction you want: into the ground, to the sky, far away behind the horizon).

Now breathe out and check if this feeling still bothers you.

How do I feel now?

Repeat as many times as you wish.

REFERENCES

History of the Selective Autophagy Research: How Did It Begin and Where Does It Stand Today?
https://www.ncbi.nlm.nih.gov/pmc/articles/PMC6971693/

From Christian de Duve to Yoshinori Ohsumi: More to autophagy than just dining at home
https://pubmed.ncbi.nlm.nih.gov/28411887/

Mitophagy: mechanisms, pathophysiological roles, and analysis
https://www.ncbi.nlm.nih.gov/pmc/articles/PMC3630798/

The Effects of Intermittent Fasting on Brain and Cognitive Function
https://www.ncbi.nlm.nih.gov/pmc/articles/PMC8470960/

S.M.A.R.T. Goals as a Weight Loss Strategy
https://dofasting.com/blog/s-m-a-r-t-goals-as-a-weight-loss-strategy/

Intermittent Fasting and Metabolic Health
https://www.ncbi.nlm.nih.gov/pmc/articles/PMC8839325/

Remodeling of the gut microbiome during Ramadan-associated intermittent fasting
https://www.ncbi.nlm.nih.gov/pmc/articles/PMC8106760/

Exploratory analysis of one versus two-day intermittent fasting protocols on the gut microbiome and plasma metabolome in adults with overweight/obesity
https://www.ncbi.nlm.nih.gov/pmc/articles/PMC9644216/

Fasting alters the gut microbiome reducing blood pressure and body weight in metabolic syndrome patients
https://www.ncbi.nlm.nih.gov/pmc/articles/PMC8010079/

Pharmacological Effects of Urolithin A and Its Role in Muscle Health and Performance: Current Knowledge and Prospects
https://www.ncbi.nlm.nih.gov/pmc/articles/PMC10609777/

Effect of Urolithin A Supplementation on Muscle Endurance and Mitochondrial Health in Older Adults
https://www.ncbi.nlm.nih.gov/pmc/articles/PMC8777576/

An increased autophagic flux contributes to the anti-inflammatory potential of urolithin A in macrophages
https://www.ncbi.nlm.nih.gov/pmc/articles/PMC5823236/

Therapeutic Potential of Mitophagy-Inducing Microflora Metabolite, Urolithin A for Alzheimer's Disease
https://www.ncbi.nlm.nih.gov/pmc/articles/PMC8617978/

Urolithin A suppresses the proliferation of endometrial cancer cells by mediating estrogen receptor-α-dependent gene expression
https://www.ncbi.nlm.nih.gov/pmc/articles/PMC5144574/

Urolithin A improves muscle strength, exercise performance, and biomarkers of mitochondrial health in a randomized trial in middle-aged adults
https://www.ncbi.nlm.nih.gov/pmc/articles/PMC9133463/

Biohacking by Dave Asprey
https://daveasprey.com/

Effect of High-Intensity Interval Training Combined with Fasting in the Treatment of Overweight and Obese Adults: A Systematic Review and Meta-Analysis
https://www.ncbi.nlm.nih.gov/pmc/articles/PMC9030367/

REHIT vs HIIT - high intensity interval training
https://www.gymandfitness.com.au/blogs/tips/rehit-vs-hiit-high-intensity-interval-training

Benefits of Self-Myofascial Release (SMR) Therapy
https://www.sportingclubofsydney.com.au/post/benefits-of-self-myofascial-release-smr-therapy

The Therapeutic Benefits of Balls and Rollers
https://haleintegrative.com/the-therapeutic-benefits-of-balls-and-rollers/

Age of Menopause and Fracture Risk in Post-Menopausal Women Randomized to Calcium + Vitamin D, Hormone Therapy, or the combination: Results from the Women's Health Initiative Clinical Trials
https://www.ncbi.nlm.nih.gov/pmc/articles/PMC5365363/

Vitamin D and calcium intake and risk of early menopause
https://www.ncbi.nlm.nih.gov/pmc/articles/PMC5445672/

Vitamin D levels and menopause-related symptoms
https://www.ncbi.nlm.nih.gov/pmc/articles/PMC4764124/

The Importance of Nutrition in Menopause and Perimenopause—A Review
https://www.ncbi.nlm.nih.gov/pmc/articles/PMC10780928/

Coenzyme Q10 Supplementation for the Reduction of Oxidative Stress: Clinical Implications in the Treatment of Chronic Diseases
https://www.ncbi.nlm.nih.gov/pmc/articles/PMC7660335/

Coenzyme Q10 in Cardiovascular and Metabolic Diseases: Current State of the Problem
https://www.ncbi.nlm.nih.gov/pmc/articles/PMC6131403/

The Paradox of Coenzyme Q10 in Aging
https://www.ncbi.nlm.nih.gov/pmc/articles/PMC6770889/

ABOUT THE AUTHOR

Carmen Thies is a dedicated midwife, nurse, and nutritionist with over a decade of experience in women's health and wellness. Drawing from her personal journey of using intermittent fasting to lose weight, maintain her desired weight, and overcome binge eating, she brings a unique blend of professional expertise and personal insight to her work.

Passionate about education and understanding the body, Carmen Thies believes in empowering women to live happy and healthy lives through knowledge and holistic wellness practices. When she's not teaching or writing, she enjoys traveling, cooking, and sharing her love of intermittent fasting with others.

THANK YOU FOR PURCHASING THIS BOOK!

I sincerely thank you for choosing "Intermittent Fasting for Women Over 50: A Comprehensive Guide to Lose Weight, Challenge Aging, Revitalize Energy, and Achieve Hormonal Balance for Lifelong Health and Confidence." I hope that you find the insights and strategies within these pages both inspiring and practical.

If you have a moment, I would greatly appreciate it if you could share your thoughts and experiences by leaving a review on Amazon. Your feedback not only helps improve my work but also assists other readers in making informed decisions about their health and wellness choices.

Thank you once again for your support. Happy reading, and here's to your health!

Made in United States
North Haven, CT
13 June 2024

53583444R10065